Genetics

IN OBSTETRICS AND GYNECOLOGY

THE AMERICAN COLLEGE OF
OBSTETRICIANS AND GYNECOLOGISTS
WOMEN'S HEALTH CARE PHYSICIANS
409 12TH STREET, SW
PO BOX 96920
WASHINGTON, DC 20090-6920

Genetics in Obstetrics and Gynecology contains current clinical practice documents published by the American College of Obstetricians and Gynecologists (ACOG) as of June 30, 2002. The information in these documents should not be viewed as establishing standards or dictating rigid rules. The guidelines are general and intended to be adapted to many different situations, taking into account the needs and resources particular to the locality, the institution, or the type of practice. Variations and innovations that improve the quality of patient care are to be encouraged rather than restricted. The purpose of these guidelines will be well served if they provide a firm basis on which local norms may be built.

The American College of Obstetricians and Gynecologists
409 12th Street, SW
PO Box 96920
Washington, DC 20090-6920

ISBN 0-915473-86-0

Copies of *Genetics in Obstetrics and Gynecology* as well as individual copies of each document in this book can be obtained from ACOG's web site (www.acog.org) and from ACOG's Resource Center; call (202) 863-2518 or e-mail resources@acog.org to order. Bulk copies also are available from ACOG's Distribution Center; call 800-762-2264 or go to sales.acog.com to order.

12345/65432

CONTENTS

Preface

The purpose of *Genetics in Obstetrics and Gynecology* is to assist obstetrician–gynecologists in understanding and applying the concepts of molecular genetics to clinical practice, research, and the provision of health care in the community. The first document, entitled "Genetics and Molecular Diagnostic Testing," also is the first document in the new ACOG series, "Technology Assessment in Obstetrics and Gynecology." This document reviews the basics of genetic testing and genetic technologies in current use. The Committee on Genetics of the American College of Obstetricians and Gynecologists (ACOG) wishes to thank Deborah A. Driscoll, MD, FACOG; Katherine D. Wenstrom, MD, FACOG; and John Williams, III, MD, FACOG, for their assistance in the development of "Genetics and Molecular Diagnostic Testing."

Genetics in Obstetrics and Gynecology contains all of the current documents issued by ACOG's Committee on Genetics as of June 30, 2002. These documents have been compiled into one volume for ease of use and reference. It is important to bear in mind that in addition to *Genetics in Obstetrics and Gynecology*, ACOG has other publications and information related to genetics for professionals, such as ACOG's *Compendium of Selected Publications* and *Guidelines for Perinatal Care,* which is published with the American Academy of Pediatrics.

As the practice of medicine evolves, so too do ACOG documents. This is particularly true for the rapidly evolving technologies and the clinical practice of genetics. ACOG will continue to update information presented here through clinical statements and recommendations that are issued periodically. As new documents are published, which may replace or supplement existing documents in *Genetics in Obstetrics and Gynecology*, they will be included in the ACOG publications section of *Obstetrics & Gynecology*. Any new genetics documents that are published after June 30, 2002, will be included in ACOG's *Compendium of Selected Publications* until an update of *Genetics in Obstetrics and Gynecology* is published.

ACOG
TECHNOLOGY ASSESSMENT
IN OBSTETRICS AND GYNECOLOGY

NUMBER 1, JULY 2002

This Technology Assessment was developed by the ACOG Committee on Genetics with the assistance of Deborah A. Driscoll, MD, FACOG; Katherine D. Wenstrom, MD, FACOG, and John Williams III, MD, FACOG. This document reflects emerging clinical and scientific advances as of the date issued and is subject to change. The information should not be construed as dictating an exclusive course of treatment or procedure to be followed. Variations in practice may be warranted based on the needs of the individual patient, resources, and limitations unique to the institution or type of practice.

THE AMERICAN COLLEGE OF OBSTETRICIANS AND GYNECOLOGISTS
WOMEN'S HEALTH CARE PHYSICIANS

Genetics and Molecular Diagnostic Testing

Knowledge of human genetics has increased dramatically in the past few decades. The genetic basis of disease and the response to therapy is rapidly being elucidated and may soon become a part of routine medical practice. A draft of the human genome was published in 2001 (1). This project produced a detailed map of the genes, markers, and other landmarks along each chromosome. It is hoped that these maps will facilitate the development of genetic screening and diagnostic tests, as well as novel therapies, technologies, and strategies for prevention. Obstetricians and gynecologists, who deal with inheritance and the genetic transmission of traits and disease on a daily basis, will be called on to incorporate genetics and recent developments in genetic testing into their medical practice. This document reviews the basics of genetic transmission and genetic technologies in current use. (See the "Glossary" for definitions of terms for genetics and molecular diagnostic testing.)

Organization of the Genome

There are 2 meters of DNA, including approximately 30,000 genes, in each human nucleus. The DNA is wrapped very compactly around basic proteins called histones to form nucleosomes, which are then organized into solenoid structures and looped around a nonhistone protein scaffold to form chromatin. As the cell enters prophase, the chromatin begins to condense until it assumes the familiar structure of metaphase chromosomes. Each chromosome is composed of densely packed nontranscribed DNA near the centromeres, called heterochromatin, and less densely packed transcribed DNA called euchromatin.

Seventy-five percent of the genome is unique, single copy DNA, and the remainder consists of various classes of repetitive DNA. Surprisingly, virtually all of the repetitive DNA and a large portion of the single copy DNA have no apparent or recognized function. Less than 10% of the genome encodes genes. The single copy DNA contains all of the genes necessary to make and sustain the organism, while the repetitive DNA contains unique markers that identify each individual and can be used to study genetic variation between individuals.

Genes

A gene is a unique series of four purine and pyrimidine bases that ultimately specifies an amino acid sequence for a polypeptide chain of a protein. The basic gene contains one or more exons, which are DNA sequences that will be transcribed into messenger RNA (mRNA), and introns (or intervening sequences), which are noncoding or nontranscribed regions that separate exons (Fig. 1). The regions upstream and downstream to the exons are called the 5′ untranslated region and the 3′ untranslated region, respectively. These regions are transcribed, but not translated (as the name implies), and they are important in gene regulation.

The processes of transcription and translation are more complex than previously recognized. The transcription of DNA to mRNA requires transcription factors. Enhancers and silencer DNA sequences located upstream or downstream of a gene can increase and decrease transcriptional activity of the gene, respectively. Transcription is initiated when the enzyme RNA polymerase II binds to the promoter, a DNA sequence upstream of a gene. RNA polymerase moves along a single strand of DNA and forms a complementary strand of mRNA. Once the mRNA is formed, a cap or chemically modified guanine nucleotide is added to the 5′ end to prevent the mRNA from being degraded, and a chain of 100–200 adenine bases (poly-A tail) is added to the 3′ end. Before the mRNA leaves the nucleus, the introns are excised by a process called gene splicing. The mature mRNA then moves to the ribosomes for translation. The protein product usually is created in a precursor form, and undergoes cleavage into a smaller active protein or combines with other polypeptides to form a larger functional protein. The protein may be further modified in the Golgi apparatus of the cell by glycosylation. Some genes contain more than one promoter in different parts of the gene or have alternative splice sites, which allows the same gene to encode different protein products.

Gene expression also is controlled by methylation of the regulatory region, which prevents gene transcription and effectively turns the gene off. Methylation serves the important function of controlling tissue-specific gene activation. The expression

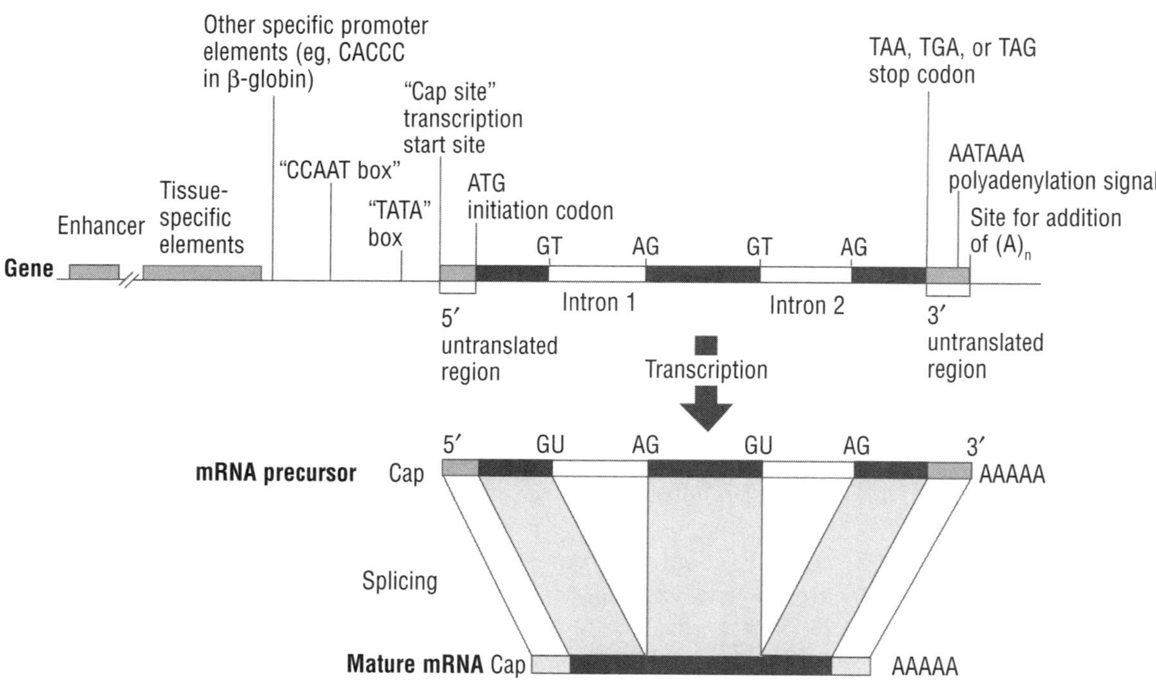

Fig. 1. Structure of a typical gene. In this example, the gene has three exons (solid dark regions) and two introns (white regions), a 5′ untranslated region and 3′ untranslated region. The intron splice donor site (GT) and the splice acceptor site (AG) identify where introns are removed in mRNA production. The upstream region (5′) contains an enhancer, tissue specific elements, and promoter elements, such as the CCAAT box and TATA box, which regulate expression. Typical locations for the translation initiation site (ATG), translation stop codons (TAA, TAG, TGA), and the polyadenylation signal (AATAAA) are shown. (Gelehrter TD, Ginsburg D, Collins FS. Principles of medical genetics. 2nd ed. Baltimore: Williams and Wilkins, 1997)

of genes that are not essential for each specific tissue type is prevented by methylation, while necessary genes remain active. For example, the globin genes are methylated in all nonerythroid tissues but are not methylated in reticulocytes, ensuring that only red blood cells produce hemoglobin. Methylation also allows the temporal control of gene expression. Parental alleles may demonstrate different patterns of methylation that are not tissue specific (see section on "Imprinting").

Many genes exist in several alternate forms called alleles. These are normal variants within the population. For example, there are several normal alleles for the genes that determine blood type and Rh status. In contrast, a mutation is an alteration in the DNA sequence that results in a change in protein structure or function, which may have adverse effects. Mutations can occur in the germline (eg, gametes) and can be transmitted from one generation to the next, or can occur only in the somatic cells and can be associated with cancer. There are many types of mutations, such as single purine or pyrimidine base substitutions (missense, nonsense), deletions and insertions of one or more bases, and visible chromosome deletions and duplications. Mutations occur infrequently in the population. The distinction between an allele and a mutation can be blurred; many normal alleles probably result from ancient mutations that either did not affect survival or conferred some selective advantage.

The vast majority (99.8%) of DNA is identical in all humans. However, minor differences that distinguish one person from another do exist. These differences, called polymorphisms, generally consist of a single nucleotide change and occur every 200 to 500 base pairs. Polymorphisms, in general, do not produce deleterious effects. Some polymorphisms may modify gene function (eg, splice variant or thymidine tract in intron 8 of the cystic fibrosis (CF) gene can influence the amount of mRNA produced). In most cases, polymorphisms are normal variants, which often are used to track the transmission of disease genes (see sections on "Restriction Fragment Length Polymorphism Analysis" and "Linkage Analysis").

When newly discovered genes are analyzed, it can be difficult to distinguish a normal allele from a polymorphism or a mutation. For example, more than 100 variations of the *BRCA1* gene, one of the major genes associated with familial breast and ovarian cancers, have been identified. It is not currently known whether all of these variations are actually mutations associated with disease, or if some could be polymorphisms or allelic variants. The ability to distinguish alleles from mutations is essential for molecular diagnosis and screening programs.

SINGLE GENE (MENDELIAN) DISORDERS

A mendelian trait or disease is determined by a single gene. Diseases caused solely by abnormalities in a single gene are relatively rare. The phenotype of many single gene disorders is influenced by modifying genes, or by the independent actions of a combination of additional genes, often with environmental influences.

Autosomal Dominant

All genes come in pairs; one copy of the gene is present on each of a pair of chromosomes. The influence of each gene in determining the phenotype is described as either dominant or recessive. If one of the genes in a pair specifies the phenotype in preference to the other gene, that gene and the trait or disease it specifies are considered to be dominant. The carrier of a gene causing an autosomal dominant disease has a 50% chance of passing on the affected gene with each conception.

The phenotype of an individual carrying a dominant gene is determined by several factors. One factor is penetrance. Penetrance indicates whether or not the mutant gene is expressed. If a dominant gene produces some kind of recognizable phenotypic expression in all individuals who carry it, it is said to have complete penetrance. A gene that is not expressed in all individuals who carry it has incomplete penetrance. For individuals, penetrance is an all-or-nothing phenomenon, but penetrance in a population can be quantitated. For example, a phenotype that is expressed in 80% of individuals who carry the gene has 80% penetrance.

Incomplete penetrance may account for some autosomal dominant diseases that appear to "skip" generations. Alternatively, the individual carrying the dominant gene may have very mild phenotypic abnormalities that have been overlooked, the disease may have a late onset, the gene carrier is either too young or died before the gene's effects were manifest, or phenotypic expression of the dominant gene could require the presence of a second mutated gene or certain epigenetic phenomena. An example of such a disease is retinoblastoma.

The degree to which a penetrant gene is expressed (the range of phenotypic features) is called expressivity. If all individuals carrying the affected gene do not have identical phenotypes, the gene has variable expressivity. Such a gene can produce a range of phenotypic features from mild to severe. An example of a disease with variable expressivity is neurofibromatosis.

Autosomal Recessive

Autosomal recessive traits or diseases occur only when both copies of the gene in question are the same. Individuals who have only one abnormal gene (heterozygotes or carriers) may have some phenotypic alteration recognized at the biochemical or cellular level, but only individuals who have two copies of the affected gene (homozygotes) have the disease. Many enzyme deficiency diseases are autosomal recessive. The enzyme level in the carrier of an abnormal recessive gene will be approximately 50% of normal, but because enzymes are made in great excess, this reduction usually is not enough to cause disease. However, the reduced enzyme level can be used for genetic screening purposes. For example, to identify carriers of Tay–Sachs disease, hexosaminidase A levels are measured. Carriers of recessive conditions that do not produce any physical or quantitative biochemical change in the heterozygote can be identified only by molecular methods (eg, Canavan disease).

The carrier of a gene causing an autosomal recessive disease usually is recognized after the birth of an affected child, after the diagnosis of an affected family member, or as the result of a genetic screening program. A couple whose child has an autosomal recessive disease has a 25% recurrence risk with each conception. The likelihood that a normal sibling of an affected child is a carrier of the gene is 2 out of 3 (one fourth of all offspring will be homozygous normal, two fourths will be heterozygote carriers, and one fourth will be homozygous abnormal; thus, 3 of 4 children will be phenotypically normal and 2 of these 3 will be carriers). Carrier children will not have affected children unless their partners are gene carriers or are affected. Because genes leading to rare autosomal recessive conditions have a low prevalence in the general population, the chance that the partner will be a gene carrier is low unless the couple is related (consanguineous). When individuals inherit two different mutated alleles that result in abnormal phenotypes, they are called compound heterozygotes. For example, an individual who inherits a ΔF508 and W1282X mutation in the CF gene has CF without expressing two identical alleles.

Co-Dominant

If the genes in a gene pair are different from each other, but both are expressed in the phenotype, they are considered to be co-dominant. For example, the genes responsible for the hemoglobinopathies are co-dominant. The individual with one hemoglobin gene directing the production of sickle hemoglobin, and the other directing the production of hemoglobin C, will produce both S and C hemoglobins. Likewise, the genes that determine blood type are co-dominant, because an individual is capable of expressing both A and B red cell antigens simultaneously.

X-Linked

X-linked diseases usually are recessive, and primarily affect men because men have only one copy of the X chromosome. Examples of X-linked recessive disorders are color blindness, hemophilia A (classical hemophilia or factor VIII deficiency), and Duchenne muscular dystrophy. Women carrying an X-linked recessive gene generally are unaffected unless unfavorable lyonization (the inactivation of one X chromosome in every cell) results in the X chromosome carrying the abnormal gene being active in the majority of cells.

When a woman carries a gene causing an X-linked recessive condition, there is a 50% chance of passing on the gene with each conception; each of her sons has a 50% chance of being affected and each of her daughters has a 50% chance of being a carrier. When a man has an X-linked disease, all of his sons will be unaffected (because they receive the Y chromosome from their father) and all of his daughters will be carriers (because they receive the affected X chromosome from their father). X-linked dominant disorders have been described, and affect females predominantly because they tend to be lethal in male offspring. An example of this is X-linked hypophosphatemia.

DUPLICATION AND DELETION SYNDROMES

A deletion refers to a region of a chromosome that is missing, while a duplication is the presence of an extra copy of a region of a chromosome. The carrier of a deletion is effectively monosomic for the genes in the missing segment, while the carrier of a duplication is trisomic for the duplicated genes. Deletions and duplications usually are described by their location (eg, duplication 4p) or by the two chromosomal break points defining the missing or extra segment (4p15.2→16.1). If the deletion is a common one, it may be defined by an eponym (eg, del 1q32-q41 also is called Van der Woude's syndrome). Terminal deletions and duplications are caused simply by chromosome breakage with loss or gain of the terminal chromosome segment. Interstitial deletions and duplications occur during prophase of meiosis when homologous chromosomes align and crossovers occur. If the chromosomes are misaligned during this process, the unaligned loop containing the mismatched segment could be deleted. Alternatively, misalignment could lead to unequal crossing over, so that one chromosome has a deletion and the other a duplication. A similar problem with meiosis can produce deletions and duplications in the offspring of individuals who are carriers of chromosome inversions. Deletions and duplications also occur as a result of malsegregation during meiosis in carriers of balanced translocations.

When a deletion or duplication is identified in a fetus or child, the parents should be tested to see if it arose de novo in their offspring or if either parent is a carrier or has a translocation. Deletions and duplications may be identified by routine or high resolution cytogenetic analysis. Microdeletions and duplications, which are too small to be detected by traditional cytogenetic techniques, can now be recognized with molecular techniques, such as fluorescence in situ hybridization (FISH) (see section on "Fluorescence In Situ Hybridization").

Chromosome deletions and duplications can result in a constellation of phenotypic abnormalities with widely varying pathophysiology or pathogenesis because the genes that are in close proximity to one another on a chromosome may have completely unrelated functions and control independent traits. Deletion syndromes usually cause more serious phenotypic and functional abnormalities than duplication syndromes. Monosomy generally has more severe consequences than trisomy.

Syndromes caused by a microdeletion involving genes physically located together in a chromosome segment are called contiguous gene deletion syndromes, and their study has yielded a great deal of information about gene location and function. Although deletions can occur in any area of any chromosome, some deletions occur more frequently than would be expected by chance alone. Several common chromosome deletion syndromes have been recognized, such as DiGeorge syndrome, which most often results from a microdeletion of the long arm of chromosome 22 (del 22q11.2). Affected individuals typically have conotruncal cardiac defects; thymus and parathyroid gland hypoplasia or aplasia; atypical facies, including short palpebral fissures, micrognathia with a short philtrum, and ear anomalies; and learning and speech difficulties. Deletions of the terminal portions of the short arms of chromosomes 4 (4 p- or Wolf-Hirschhorn syndrome) and 5 (5 p- or cri du chat syndrome) also occur more frequently than would be expected by chance alone.

NONMENDELIAN PATTERNS OF INHERITANCE

Hereditary Unstable DNA

Mendel's first law states that genes are passed unchanged from parent to progeny. Barring the occurrence of new mutations, this law still applies to many genes or traits. However, it is now known that certain genes are inherently unstable, and their size and, consequently, their function may be altered as they are transmitted from parent to child. These genes generally contain a region of triplet repeats, such as $(CGG)_n$. The number of triplet repeats in gametes can increase as meiosis is completed prior to fertilization. If the number of triplet repeats reaches a critical level, the gene containing the triplets becomes methylated and is turned off, resulting in phenotypic abnormalities. Some triplet regions expand only during female meiosis, while others can expand when transmitted by either parent. Some triplet regions have been passed from parent to child for many generations without expansion, for unknown reasons.

An example of a genetic disease caused by such triplet repeats is fragile X syndrome. Fragile X syndrome is the most common form of all familial mental retardation, accounting for 4–8% of all individuals with mental retardation in all ethnic and racial groups. Affected individuals have mild to severe mental retardation, autistic behavior, attention deficit hyperactivity disorder, speech and language problems, a narrow face with a large jaw, long prominent ears, and macro-orchidism (in postpubertal males). Some children also have seizures. The incidence of the full fragile X syndrome generally is quoted as 1 per 1,500 males and 1 per 2,500 females.

Until recently, fragile X syndrome was diagnosed using a cytogenetic technique. Cells were cultured in a folate deficient medium, which resulted in fragile sites identified cytogenetically as nonstaining gaps or constrictions on the long arm of the X chromosome (Xq27-28). This technique was unreliable for carrier testing, and less than half the cells from affected males manifested the fragile site. Fortunately, the fragile X gene can now be directly examined using molecular techniques (see section on "Trinucleotide Repeat Analysis").

The fragile X mutation is now known to be a region of unstable DNA in the X chromosome. The region is best described as a series of CGG (cytosine–guanine–guanine) repeats at Xq27. The number of repeats and the degree of methylation determines whether or not an individual is affected. Individuals carrying 2–49 repeats are phenotypically normal.

Individuals carrying 50–199 repeats are phenotypically normal but have a premutation, which can expand as it is passed on to their offspring, who would then be affected. Those with more than 200 repeats have the full mutation and, if methylation occurs, usually are affected. However, not all individuals carrying the full mutation are mentally retarded. Phenotypic variability results from lyonization (in females) and mosaicism for the size of the expansion, the degree of methylation, or both during mitosis in the zygote. Therefore, the phenotype cannot be predicted by analysis of either the parental gene or fetal cells.

The number of repeats usually remains stable when the gene is transmitted by a male. However, when the gene passes through female meiosis, it can expand. The risk of expansion generally correlates with the number of repeats in the premutation. Premutations with 100 or more repeats expand on transmission 100% of the time. The risk of expansion of mutations with 50–99 repeats increases proportionally with expansion size. If a female carries a premutation, which then increases in size as she transmits it to her offspring, it is possible for her to have a child with fragile X syndrome even though she is unaffected and has no family history of mental retardation.

The number of CGG repeats and the methylation status of the gene can be determined using restriction endonuclease digestion and Southern blot analysis (see section on "Trinucleotide Repeat Analysis"). It is now apparent that triplet repeat expansion is responsible for a number of primarily neurologic diseases, such as myotonic dystrophy, Huntington's chorea, and Friedreich's ataxia. The expansion of triplet repeats is an important mechanism of genetic disease, and is likely to play an important part in diseases for which preconceptional counseling and prenatal diagnosis may be considered.

Imprinting

Another tenet of mendelian genetics is that gene function is not influenced by the sex of the parent transmitting the gene. In contrast to this rule, it is now apparent that the function of certain genes is altered by the sex of the parent from whom they were inherited, by a process known as "imprinting." Imprinting is a mechanism for epigenetic control of gene expression; that is, it changes the phenotype without permanently altering the genotype. An imprinted gene is inherited in an inactivated (transcriptionally silent) state, as the result of methylation of the promoter region. The extent of the imprinting, and thus the degree of inactivation, is determined by the sex of the transmitting parent.

When a gene is inherited in an imprinted or inactivated state, gene function is necessarily directed entirely by the active co-gene inherited from the other parent. It appears that imprinting exerts an effect in part by controlling the dosage of specific genes. Certain important genes appear to be monoallelic; that is, under normal circumstances only one member of the gene pair is functional (as opposed to most of the genes in the genome, which are biallelic). Only a fraction of human genes are imprinted. With imprinted genes, however, normal development occurs only when both a paternally derived and a maternally derived copy of the gene is present.

Imprinting was first recognized in association with genetic disease. Two very distinct genetic diseases with dissimilar phenotypes were discovered to be associated with the same chromosomal deletion, at 15q11-13. One of the diseases is Prader-Willi syndrome, which is characterized by obesity; hyperphagia; short stature; small hands, feet, and external genitalia; and mild mental retardation. The other disorder is Angelman's syndrome, which includes normal stature and weight, severe mental retardation, absent speech, seizure disorder, ataxia and jerky arm movements, and paroxysms of inappropriate laughter. Cytogenetic analysis has confirmed that both diseases are associated with the same deletion. If the maternally derived chromosome 15 is deleted, the result is Angelman's syndrome; if the paternally derived chromosome 15 is deleted, the result is Prader-Willi syndrome. Furthermore, a deletion is not required to produce the phenotype. If an individual has two normal intact copies of chromosome 15, but both came from the man (see section on "Uniparental Disomy"), the phenotype is consistent with Angelman's syndrome, because the maternal contribution is missing. Likewise, two complete copies of chromosome 15 of maternal origin produces Prader-Willi syndrome. Studies of the methylation patterns in individuals with the 15q11-13 deletion have shown that differential methylation (imprinting) is responsible for these observed phenotypic differences.

Several clinical examples from obstetrics illustrate the developmental importance of imprinting. Complete hydatidiform mole, which has an exclusively paternally derived diploid chromosome complement, is characterized by the abundant growth of placental tissue, but no fetal structures. Conversely, ovarian teratoma, which has a maternally derived diploid chromosome complement, is characterized by the growth of various fetal tissues, but no placental structures. Triploidy, characterized by a conceptus with three complete haploid chromosome complements (69 chromosomes), has two distinct phenotypes. If the extra haploid chromosome complement comes from the man, the embryo will be lost early in gestation and the placenta will be large and cystic, and severe early onset preeclampsia is likely to develop; if the extra chromosome complement comes from the woman, the fetus will be anomalous and the placenta will be extremely small. These observations confirm that both the paternally derived and maternally derived imprinted genes must be present for normal fetal development to occur.

Uniparental Disomy

Uniparental disomy is a situation in which both members of one pair of chromosomes are inherited from one parent. Every gene on each of the chromosomes in question will have come from one parent. This usually occurs as the result of "correction" of a trisomic zygote by loss of a chromosome. When a conceptus with three copies of a chromosome loses one chromosome and retains the two chromosomes transmitted by the other parent, this results in heterodisomy (inheritance of two different homologous chromosomes from one parent). Less frequently, "rescue" of a monosomic conceptus with only one chromosome from one parent may occur by duplication of the chromosome during mitosis producing a cell with two copies of the same chromosome or uniparental isodisomy. For some chromosomes, uniparental disomy can result in functional or developmental fetal abnormalities, particularly if imprinting of the genes on that chromosome exists. Recent studies have demonstrated clinically significant uniparental disomy for chromosomes 6, 7, 11, 14, and 15. Uniparental disomy has no effect on the majority of chromosomes.

Mitochondrial Inheritance

Every human cell contains hundreds of mitochondria. Because each mitochondrian contains its own genome and associated replication systems, each behaves as a virtually autonomous organism. The human oocyte contains approximately 100,000 mitochondria in the cytoplasm and mitochondrial DNAs. In contrast, a sperm contains only 100 mitochondria, which are selectively eliminated during fertilization. Therefore, mitochondria are inherited exclusively from the woman. Because mitochondria contain genetic information, mitochondrial inheritance allows the transmission of genes directly from the woman to her offspring without the possibility of recombination.

If a mutation occurs in the mitochondrial DNA, it may segregate into a daughter cell during cell division and thus be propagated. Over time, the percentage of mutant mitochondrial DNAs in different cell lines can drift towards either normal or pure mutant. If an oocyte containing largely mutant mitochondrial DNAs is fertilized, the offspring might have a mitochondrial disease. Several mitochondrial genetic diseases have been described. These include myoclonic epilepsy with ragged red fibers (MERRF), Leber's hereditary optic neuropathy, Kearns–Sayre syndrome, Leigh syndrome (ataxia, hypotonia, spasticity, and optic abnormalities), and pigmentary retinopathy.

Germline Mosaicism

Some cytogenetically normal individuals have mosaicism (the presence of two or more populations of cells with different characteristics within one tissue or organ) confined to their gonads. Gonadal or germline mosaicism can arise as the result of a mitotic error occurring in the zygote; if the error occurs in cells destined to become the gonad, a portion of the germ cells may be abnormal. Because spermatogonia and oogonia continue to divide throughout fetal development, gonadal mosaicism also could occur as the result of a meiotic error in the dividing germ cells of the embryo. Germline mosaicism may explain the occurrence of a "new" (not previously occurring in a family) autosomal dominant mutation causing a disease, such as achondroplasia or osteogenesis imperfecta, or a new X-linked disease, such as Duchenne muscular dystrophy. It also explains the recurrence of such diseases in more than one offspring in a previously unaffected family. Because of the potential for germline mosaicism, the recurrence risk after the birth of a child with a disease caused by a new mutation is approximately 6%.

Multifactorial and Polygenic Inheritance

Polygenic traits are determined by the combined effects of many genes; multifactorial traits are determined by multiple genes and environmental factors. It is now believed that the majority of inherited traits are multifactorial or polygenic. Traits determined by single genes and transmitted by strict mendelian inheritance, without the contribution of modifier genes, are probably relatively rare. Birth defects caused by multifactorial or polygenic inheritance are recognized by their tendency to recur in families, but not according to a mendelian inheritance pattern. Other characteristics that distinguish multifactorial traits from those with other inheritance patterns are listed in the box. When counseling couples regarding their offspring's risk of a familial multifactorial trait, it is important to consider the affected relative's degree of relatedness to the fetus, not the parents.

Multifactorial Inheritance

1. The disorder is familial, but there is no apparent pattern of inheritance.
2. The risk to first-degree relatives is the square root of the population risk.
3. The risk is sharply lower for second-degree relatives.
4. The recurrence risk is higher if more than one family member is affected.
5. The risk is higher if the defect is more severe (ie, the recurrence risk for bilateral cleft lip is higher than for unilateral cleft lip).
6. If the defect is more common in one sex, the recurrence risk is higher if the affected individual is of the less commonly affected sex.

The empiric recurrence risk for first-degree relatives (the fetus's parents or siblings) usually is quoted as 2–3%, but the risk declines exponentially with successively more distant relationships. Multifactorial traits generally fall into one of the three following categories: 1) continuously variable, 2) threshold, or 3) complex disorders.

Continuously variable traits have a normal distribution in the general population. By convention, abnormality is defined as a trait or measurement greater than two standard deviations above or below the population mean. These are typically measurable or quantitative traits like height or head size, and are believed to result from the individually small effects of many genes combined with environmental factors. Such traits tend to be less extreme in the offspring of affected individuals, because of the statistical principle of regression to the mean.

Threshold traits do not appear until a certain threshold of liability is exceeded. Factors creating liability to the malformation are assumed to be continuously distributed in the population; only individuals who are at the extreme of this distribution exceed the threshold and have the trait or defect. The phenotypic abnormality is thus an all or none phenomenon. Individuals in high-risk families have enough abnormal genes or environmental influences that their liability is close to the threshold; for unknown reasons, some factor or factors increases the liability for certain family members still further and the threshold is crossed, resulting in the defect. Cleft lip and palate and pyloric stenosis are examples of threshold traits.

Certain threshold traits have a predilection for one gender, indicating that males and females have a different liability threshold. When a family includes an affected member who is the less frequently affected sex, this indicates that even more abnormal genes or environmental influences are present, and the affected individual (and possibly the family) has a more extreme position in the normal distribution of predisposing factors. The affected person's first-degree relatives (eg, their siblings) have a higher liability for that particular trait. For example, pyloric stenosis is more common in males. If a girl is born with pyloric stenosis, this indicates that she or her parents have even more abnormal genes or predisposing factors than usually are necessary to produce pyloric stenosis. After the birth of a girl with pyloric stenosis, the recurrence risk for her siblings or for her future children will be higher than expected; male siblings or offspring will have the highest liability because they are the most susceptible sex and they will inherit more than the usual number of predisposing genes.

The recurrence risk for threshold traits also is higher if the defect is severe, again indicating the presence of more abnormal genes or influences. For example, the recurrence risk after the birth of a child with bilateral cleft lip and palate is 8%, compared with only 4% after unilateral cleft lip without cleft palate.

Complex disorders of adult life are traits in which many genes determine an individual's susceptibility to environmental factors, with disease resulting from the most unfavorable combination of both. This category includes common diseases, such as heart disease and hypertension. These disorders usually are familial and behave as threshold traits but with a very strong environmental influence. The genetic mechanisms of many common adult diseases have not yet been elucidated, although several associated genes have been identified. In some cases, the identity of the associated gene provides a clue to the pathogenesis of the disease; in others, the related gene may simply be used as a disease marker. Premature cardiovascular diseases, for example, are associated with the gene for apolipoprotein E, a gene that likely influences the pathology of the disease. In contrast, the association of type 1 diabetes with HLA-DR3/4 is less clear.

MOLECULAR DIAGNOSTIC TESTING

Advances in our understanding of the molecular basis of inherited disorders have led to the development of DNA-based tests, which may be used for the confirmation of a diagnosis, prenatal diagnosis, and carrier testing. Molecular diagnostic testing is now widely available for a number of single gene disorders, such as Tay–Sachs disease, Canavan disease, sickle cell disease, CF, muscular dystrophies, and fragile X syndrome. Molecular-cytogenetic testing has been developed for the detection of chromosomal abnormalities, including aneuploidy and submicroscopic deletions and duplications.

DNA can be obtained from many sources, including blood lymphocytes, skin, hair, cheek cells, and paraffin tissue blocks. Most diagnostic laboratories prefer either blood samples or buccal swabs for DNA testing. Cultured amniocytes, chorionic villi, and fetal blood are used for prenatal DNA testing of the fetus.

MUTATION DETECTION

Once a gene has been cloned and mutations have been identified, direct testing for the mutation is possible. This is the most accurate diagnostic method. Direct mutation tests usually are performed by commercial and hospital-based laboratories for common mutations, which are well characterized and account for the majority of cases. In some cases, the mutations are unique to a specific ethnicity. For example, two specific mutations in the aspartoacylase gene account for 97% of the mutations that cause Canavan disease in the Ashkenazi Jewish population. For some genetic disorders, the mutations are unique or specific to an individual family; therefore, mutation testing may not be routinely provided by a commercial laboratory. In these cases, there may be only one or two academic or hospital laboratories in the country that offer the testing. (This information is provided by GeneTests, a genetic testing resource web site at www.genetests.org.) In general, initial screening of a gene for mutations usually takes place in research laboratories under approved protocols and is not practical for diagnostic testing. Once a mutation has been identified, it may be possible to offer diagnostic or carrier testing to individuals at risk.

There are a variety of methods available for detecting mutations. The methodology usually is determined by the nature of the specific mutation. Allele specific oligonucleotide hybridization and restriction fragment length polymorphisms analysis frequently are used to detect point mutations. Southern blot analysis and polymerase chain reaction (PCR) often are used to detect gene deletions associated with disorders such as Duchenne muscular dystrophy and spinal muscular atrophy. A combination of PCR and Southern blot analysis are used to determine the number of trinucleotide repeats for disorders such as fragile X syndrome and myotonic dystrophy.

Southern Blot Analysis

Southern blot analysis provides a basis for studying genetic disorders at the DNA level. This procedure, named after its inventor E. M. Southern, separates DNA fragments according to size and allows the identification of specific DNA fragments using radiolabeled DNA probes.

The steps to prepare a Southern blot are shown in Figure 2. First, DNA is extracted from nucleated cells (leukocytes, trophoblasts, or amniocytes) or tissue, and digested into small pieces with a restriction enzyme. Then, the DNA is loaded into an agarose gel, an electric current is applied, and DNA fragments migrate down the gel according to size (smaller fragments move faster). The DNA contained within the agarose gel is still double stranded and

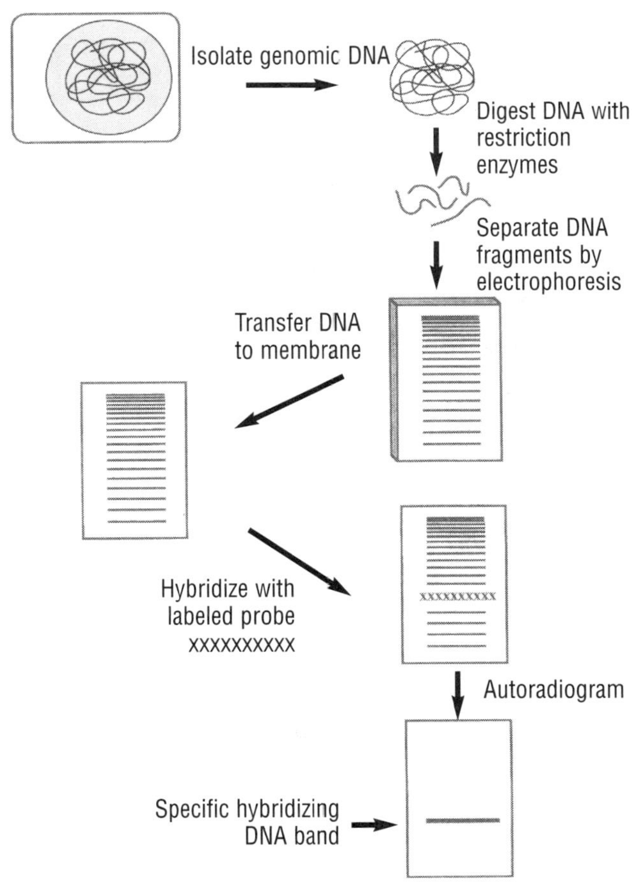

Fig. 2. Southern blot analysis. (Jameson JL. Principles of molecular medicine. Totowa, NJ: Humana Press, 1998:16)

must be denatured by alkali treatment into single-stranded pieces and then transferred to a nitrocellulose or nylon membrane. The membrane contains many thousands of fixed DNA fragments. Specific DNA fragments can be detected using a DNA probe labeled with a radionuclide, such as ^{32}P, although nonradioactive substances such as biotin–avidin may be used. The probes may be complementary DNA (cDNA), genomic DNA (exons, introns, or regulatory regions), or short pieces of single-stranded DNA called oligonucleotides, which usually range in size from 20 to 50 base pairs. The DNA probe will hybridize only with DNA fragments on the blot that are complementary. To visualize the DNA fragment, the blot is exposed to X-ray film at -70°C, a process called autoradiography. The film is developed, and the presence or absence of DNA bands or fragments can be determined.

Polymerase Chain Reaction

The development of the PCR has greatly simplified DNA analysis and shortened laboratory time. Polymerase chain reaction allows the exponential amplification of the targeted gene or DNA sequence. Only minute quantities of DNA, typically 0.1–1 μg, are necessary for PCR. DNA can be amplified from a single cell. One important prerequisite of PCR, which is not required for Southern blot analysis, is that the sequence of the gene, or at least the borders of the region of DNA to be amplified, must be known.

The PCR procedure has three steps (Fig. 3). First, DNA is denatured by heating to render it single stranded. Second, the PCR primers (primer A and B), which are short pieces of DNA (oligonucleotides) 20–30 base pairs in length exactly complementary to the ends of each piece of the double-stranded DNA to be amplified, anneal to their complementary regions of the DNA. Third, synthesis of the complementary strand of DNA occurs in the presence of the enzyme Taq polymerase and nucleotides triphosphates (dATP, dCTP, dGTP, and dTTP). The reaction cycle of denaturation, annealing, and extension is repeated 25–30 times to produce millions of copies of DNA.

Typically, fragments several kilobases (kb) in size can be amplified, but sequences up to 10 kb have been successfully amplified. The exact cycling parameters and conditions for PCR must be determined empirically for each set of primers. Polymerase chain reaction is very sensitive; therefore, extreme care must be taken to avoid amplification of contaminant DNA from aerosolized secretions or sloughed skin cells. These precautions are particularly important when DNA from a single cell is being amplified.

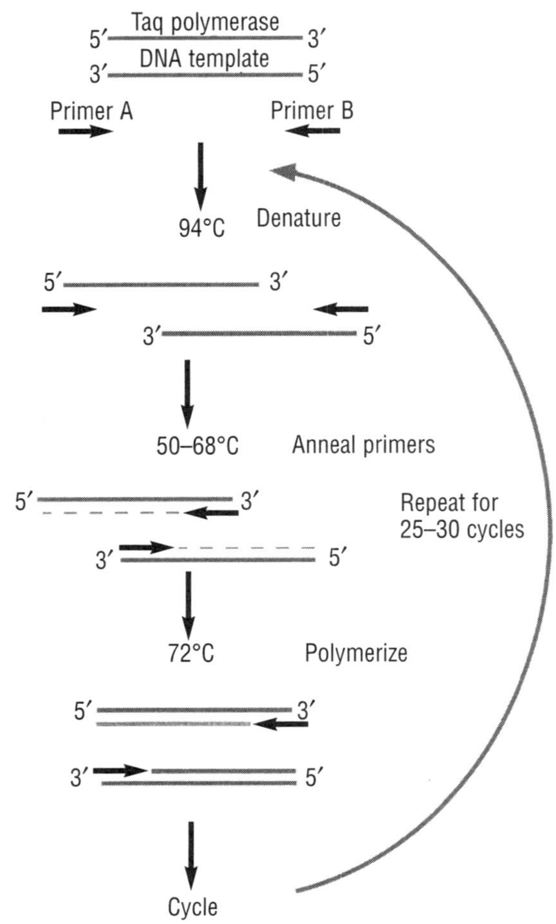

Fig. 3. Polymerase chain reaction. (Jameson JL. Principles of molecular medicine. Totowa, NJ: Humana Press, 1998:15)

Restriction Fragment Length Polymorphism Analysis

Restriction fragment length polymorphism analysis can be used when a mutation either creates or destroys a restriction endonuclease site. To detect the mutation, DNA around the site of the mutation is amplified by the PCR, incubated with the appropriate restriction enzyme, and analyzed by agarose gel electrophoresis. When a mutation creates a new restriction site, two DNA fragments will be detected if the mutation is present (Fig. 4A). An individual without the mutation will demonstrate a single fragment. This method frequently is used for the prenatal genetic diagnosis of sickle cell disease. Sickle cell disease is caused by a single base pair substitution (adenine to thymidine) in codon 6 of the β-subunit of hemoglobin, which results in the loss of the MstII restriction site. Individuals with sickle cell disease are homozygous for this mutation.

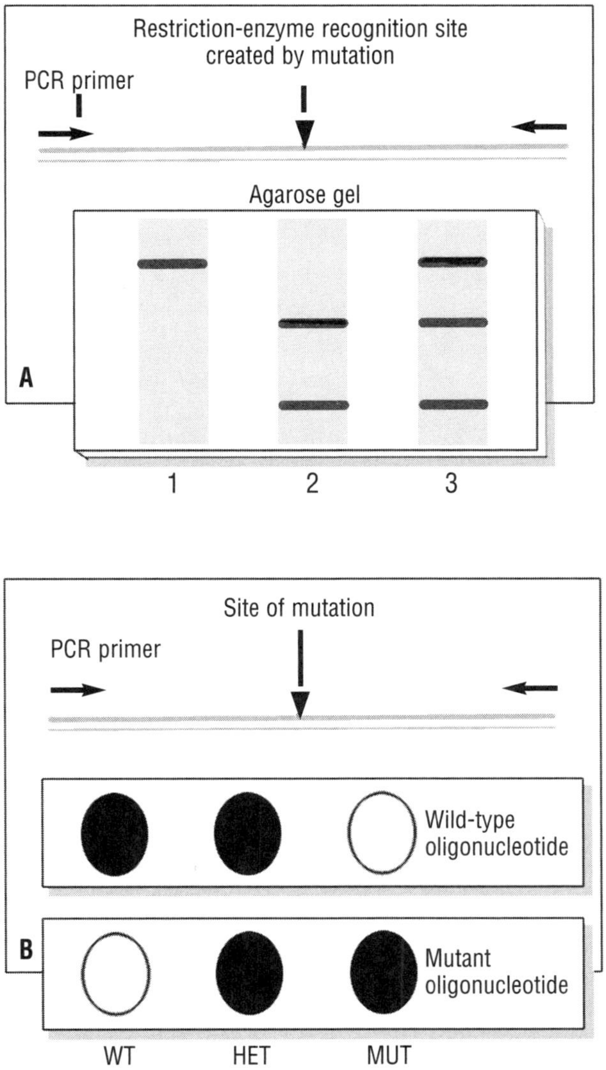

Fig. 4. Mutation detection. **(A)** Restriction fragment length polymorphism (RFLP) analysis. The region of DNA surrounding the mutation is amplified by specific PCR primers, digested with a restriction enzyme, and analyzed by agarose-gel electrophoresis. In this example, the mutation creates a new restriction site. Individuals homozygous for the mutation have two DNA fragments (Lane 2) while an individual with two normal copies has one single fragment (Lane 1). A heterozygous individual has one normal uncut fragment and two cut fragments (Lane 3). **(B)** Allele-specific oligonucleotide (ASO) hybridization. The amplified DNA from an individual homozygous for the mutation only hybridizes to the mutant oligonucleotide (MUT) whereas a heterozygous individual (HET) hybridizes to both the normal (wild-type) and the mutant. A normal individual will only hybridize to the normal oligonucleotide (WT). (Korf B. Molecular diagnosis. N Engl J Med 1995;332:1500.)

Allele Specific Oligonucleotide Hybridization (Dot Blot)

Allele specific oligonucleotide hybridization (dot blot) frequently is used to detect point mutations. A segment of DNA surrounding the mutation is amplified by PCR and then an aliquot is spotted onto a filter membrane. The membrane is hybridized with an oligonucleotide probe specific for the normal sequence and one specific for the mutation. A positive hybridization signal is detected only when the sequence of the PCR product on the membrane is complementary to the sequence of the oligonucleotide. For example, testing an individual who is heterozygous for the mutant allele will reveal a positive hybridization signal with both the normal sequence and the mutant oligonucleotide probe. DNA from individuals homozygous for the mutation will only hybridize to the mutant oligonucleotide (Fig. 4B). This technique is used for the detection of point mutations for many single gene disorders, including CF, Tay–Sachs disease, Gaucher's disease, Canavan disease, and sickle cell disease.

Deletion Analysis

Intragenic deletions can be detected by PCR or Southern blot analysis or both. Polymerase chain reaction can be used to determine the absence or presence of exons within a gene. A sample of DNA is amplified by PCR and then the PCR products are analyzed by gel electrophoresis, stained with ethidium bromide to detect the absence or presence of DNA fragments (Fig. 5). The absence of a DNA fragment indicates the presence of a deletion. This method is used routinely for diagnostic and prenatal testing for Duchenne muscular dystrophy, an X-linked disorder. Approximately 60% of patients with Duchenne muscular dystrophy have intragenic deletions in the dystrophin gene and the majority of these can be detected by PCR. Most laboratories use a multiplex strategy to examine multiple exons in one PCR. However, PCR is not useful to determine carrier status in the mothers of affected males. This requires Southern blot analysis with cDNA probes from the dystrophin gene and scanning densitometry to assess gene dosage. Testing of females at risk to be carriers based on their family history is less reliable when an affected relative is not available for DNA testing. Dosage analysis also can be used to test male patients with Duchenne muscular dystrophy with a negative result by multiplex PCR to detect duplications within the dystrophin gene, which occur in approximately 6% of patients with Duchenne muscular dystrophy.

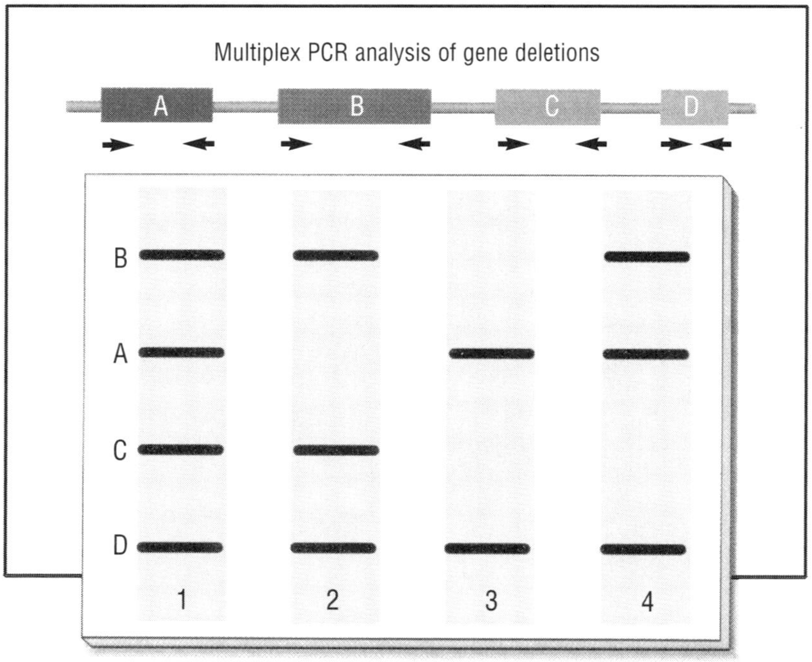

Fig. 5. Multiplex gene deletion analysis. Exons A–D are simultaneously amplified with 4 sets of PCR primers. When an exon is deleted, the DNA fragment is absent. In lane 2 exon A is absent, in lane 3 exons B and C, and in lane 4 exon C. Lane 1 shows no evidence of a deletion; all 4 DNA products are present. (Korf B. Molecular diagnosis. N Engl J Med 1995; 332:1219. Copyright © 1995 Massachusetts Medical Society. All rights reserved.)

Linkage Analysis

When the location of a gene is known but the gene has not yet been characterized, or when the mutations have not been identified, linkage analysis may be performed to predict the likelihood that a relative or fetus has inherited a disease-causing gene within an at-risk family. Linkage analysis requires that 1) at least two generations of family members, including affected individuals, are available and willing to be tested, and 2) highly polymorphic markers such as restriction fragment length polymorphisms, or short tandem repeat polymorphisms close to or within the gene are available. These polymorphic markers result from normal genetic variation and are not disease causing but may be used to track the inheritance of genetic diseases within families. The closer a marker is to a gene, the higher the likelihood that the marker and gene are transmitted or inherited together (linkage). The accuracy of linkage analysis depends on the correct diagnosis, the informativeness of the markers within the family, and the distance between the marker and the disease-causing gene. Markers closest to or within a gene are less likely to undergo recombination and will provide the most accurate prediction. Although linkage analysis is less accurate than direct mutation detection, under the specified circumstances it may provide families with helpful information.

TRINUCLEOTIDE REPEAT ANALYSIS

The detection of trinucleotide repeat expansions, associated with diseases such as fragile X syndrome, myotonic dystrophy, and Huntington's disease, often requires a combination of PCR and Southern blot analysis (Fig. 6). The size of normal alleles, premutation alleles, and, in some cases, full mutations can be determined by using PCR. However, full mutations associated with a large expansion (eg, >200 repeats in fragile X syndrome) may need to be detected using Southern blot analysis. It also is used to assess the methylation status in fragile X patients and pregnancies with the full mutation. The repeat region not only expands to more than 200 repeats but also becomes hypermethylated in affected individuals. DNA is digested with restriction enzymes including a methylation-sensitive enzyme such as BsshII, gel electrophoresed, and hybridized with a DNA probe from the repeat region of the fragile X gene (FMR-1).

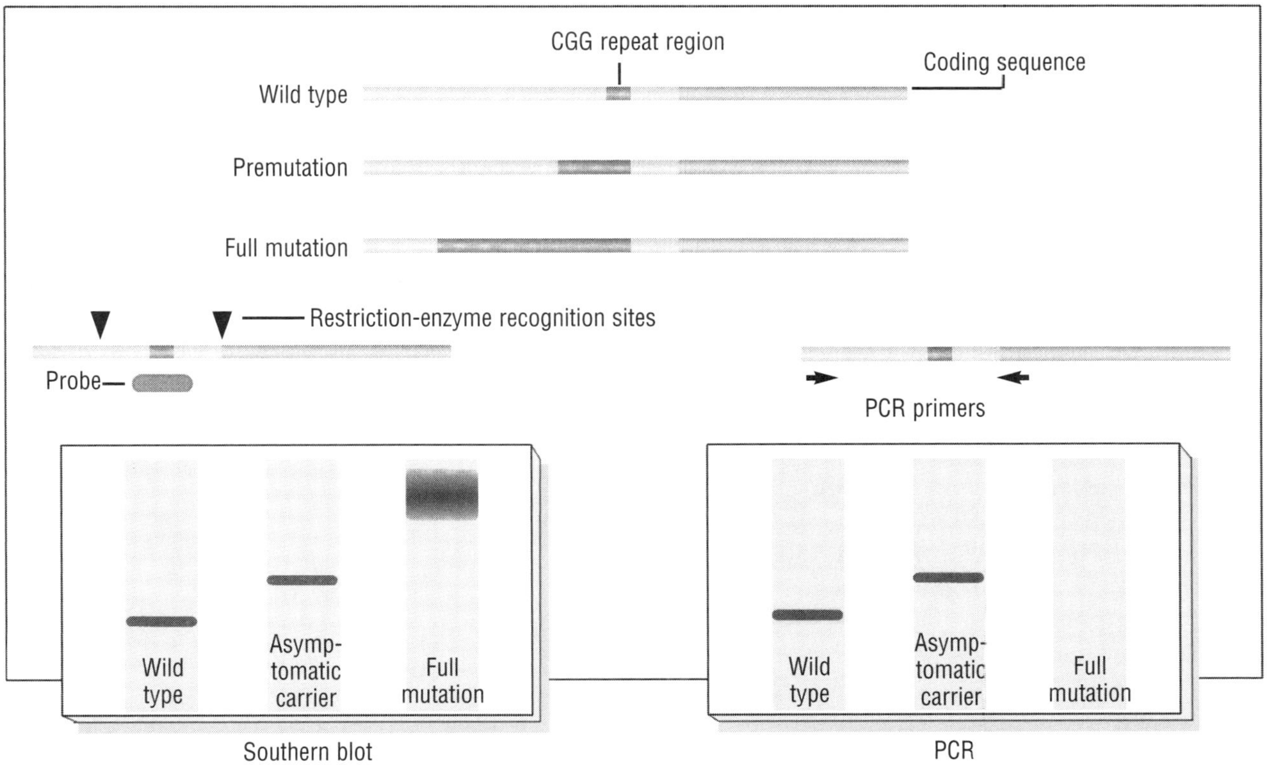

Fig. 6. Trinucleotide repeat analysis by PCR and Southern blot. A region of DNA containing the CGG repeat is amplified and the product is analyzed on an agarose gel. The DNA fragment from a carrier with a premutation is larger because of the expanded number of repeats. Sometimes the expansion is so large that the DNA fails to amplify and the number of repeats cannot be detected using PCR. In this case, a Southern blot is performed (left panel) and the DNA from an individual with a full mutation appears as a much larger band. (Korf B. Molecular diagnosis. N Engl J Med 1995;332:1501. Copyright © 1995 Massachusetts Medical Society. All rights reserved.)

FLUORESCENCE IN SITU HYBRIDIZATION

Fluorescence in situ hybridization (FISH) is performed on either metaphase chromosome preparations from cultured lymphocytes, amniocytes, or villi, or interphase nuclei from blood, tissue, chorionic villi, or amniotic fluid. After the chromosomes or nuclei are fixed on a microscope slide, they are hybridized with a fluorochrome-labeled DNA probe specific for a particular region of a chromosome. The probe will hybridize to complementary DNA sequences that can be visualized using a fluorescence microscope. Fluorescence in situ hybridization is used as an adjunct to routine cytogenetic analysis for the detection of submicroscopic chromosome deletions and duplications. These deletions and duplications often are several 1,000 base pairs but are too small to be detected by conventional cytogenetics. DNA probes have been developed for the common deletion and duplication syndromes (Table 1). It also may be used to identify or confirm the presence of a subtle chromosomal rearrangement (eg, translocation) or characterize a marker chromosome. Fluorescence in situ hybridization of interphase nuclei is used prenatally for the rapid detection of common aneuploidies, such as trisomy 21. However, this is generally reserved for cases where confirmation of a chromosomal abnormality may influence a couple's reproductive options or obstetric management.

Table 1. Microdeletion Syndromes

Syndrome	Chromosome Deletion
Aniridia/Wilm's tumor	11p13
Angelman's	15q11-13
DiGeorge/velocardiofacial	22q11.2
Langer-Giedion	8q24
Miller-Dieker	17p13.3
Prader-Willi	15q11-13
Smith-Magenis	17p11.2
Williams	7q11.23

Comparative Genomic Hybridization

Comparative genomic hybridization is a relatively new DNA-based cytogenetic technique to identify subtle chromosome deletions and duplications that have not been detected using traditional cytogenetic methods. To accomplish this, DNA from a patient is labeled with a green fluorochrome and normal control DNA is labeled with a red fluorochrome, which can be visualized with a fluorescence microscope. The DNA is hybridized to normal metaphase chromosomes. Wherever a chromosome region is duplicated, the metaphase chromosome will hybridize with the excess green-labeled DNA and appear green. Conversely, deletions will appear red. Clinically, comparative genomic hybridization is primarily used to detect cytogenetic changes in tumors but, it also has been used to identify subtle unbalanced translocations, the origin of marker or supernumerary chromosomes, and intrachromosomal duplications.

Microarray Technology

DNA chip technology is a high throughput method used primarily to study gene expression. Miniature arrays of cDNA clones are spotted onto a glass slide and hybridized with labeled cDNA prepared from the tissue of interest. If a gene is strongly expressed in the tissue, the hybridization signal will be intense. This technique can analyze the gene expression of thousands of genes at one time. In the future, oligonucleotide arrays also may be used to search for gene mutations and polymorphisms. Chips containing gene specific oligonucleotides matching normal and single nucleotides substitution sequences are hybridized with fluorescent-labeled DNA. Improvements in chip technology will enable whole genome expression screening as well as improved mutation detection in the future.

Indications for Molecular Testing

A variety of molecular diagnostic tests are available to determine whether an individual or fetus has inherited a disease-causing gene mutation. In general, testing is offered to individuals or couples identified as being at risk for a genetic disorder based on their family history, medical history, or ethnicity. Determination of an individual's carrier status for a genetic disorder provides a more accurate estimate of their risk of having an affected offspring and allows an individual or couple to consider prenatal testing options. This information also may assist couples with their reproductive decisions. Furthermore, it can identify other family members or relatives at risk for the disorder or at risk for being a carrier.

Molecular testing also may be used in clinical and prenatal situations to confirm a diagnosis. For example, screening for CF mutations may determine whether an infertile male with congenital bilateral absence of the vas deferens is a CF carrier. Prenatal molecular testing for some genetic disorders may be offered when a congenital anomaly is identified antenatally. For example, FISH for the 22q11.2 deletion may establish a cause when a conotruncal cardiac defect is detected by ultrasonography. Establishing an etiology enables clinicians to provide couples with accurate genetic risk assessments, prognostic information, and recommendations for obstetric and neonatal management.

Prior to diagnostic and carrier testing for genetic disorders, patients should be informed of the natural history of the disorder and current therapy, the inheritance and their risk of inheriting or transmitting the gene, benefits and limitations of testing, and the implications of negative and positive results. Preconceptional and prenatal testing also should include a discussion of reproductive options including prenatal testing, adoption, donor programs, and termination of pregnancy. Written informed consent should be obtained from all individuals undergoing genetic screening. Patients should understand that molecular testing is voluntary and that every effort will be made to ensure confidentiality of their medical records and test results.

Accuracy and Limitations of Molecular Testing

Direct detection of a point mutation, deletion, or duplication is the most accurate test. However, the accuracy of molecular diagnosis also is dependent on an accurate diagnosis. If an affected relative is not available to identify the presence of a mutation or if medical records are not available to confirm the diagnosis, this may decrease the accuracy of testing for a specific mutation and for the suspected genetic disorder.

One of the limitations of molecular diagnostic testing is test sensitivity. There are a number of factors that determine the ability to detect mutations. Many genetic disorders result from a variety of genetic alterations. For example, more than 800 mutations have been reported in patients with CF. The mutation detection rates for many genetic disorders, including neurofibromatosis, CF, and hemophilia, are less than 100%. Therefore, the absence of a mutation does not exclude the possibility that an individual may be a carrier. Furthermore, there may be ethnic differences in the detection rates; 97% of CF mutations have been identified in the Ashkenazi Jewish population while only 30% in Asian Americans. The incidence and carrier risk for some genetic disorders also is dependent on ethnicity and has led to the current recommendations for carrier screening for specific genetic disorders. Differences in test sensitivity and the prevalence of mutations must be considered for each individual genetic disorder and discussed with the patient prior to testing. Disease prevalence and test sensitivity should be taken into account in future recommendations for molecular-based carrier testing.

Another limitation to molecular testing is genetic heterogeneity. In some cases, there may be more than one gene or chromosomal locus responsible for a genetic disorder. For example, at least two genes have been identified that cause tuberous sclerosis, an autosomal dominant disorder. Conversely, mutations in a single gene can cause different phenotypes. For example, mutations in fibroblast growth factor receptor 3 (FGFR3) are associated with several types of skeletal disorders, including achondroplasia, hypochondroplasia, thanatophoric dysplasia, and with craniosynostosis (eg, Crouzon's disease, coronal synostosis).

In some diseases, the identification of a genetic mutation cannot precisely predict the phenotype because of reduced penetrance or phenotypic variability or both. For example, 85% of women with a *BRCA1* mutation develop breast cancer during their lifetime; therefore, the finding of a *BRCA1* mutation indicates a strong predisposition to breast cancer but it does not indicate which women with the mutation will develop a malignancy. Some genetic disorders are highly variable even within families with the same mutation. Therefore, it may only be possible to provide patients with a description of the natural history of the disorder and an estimate of the frequency of specific features in patients with similar mutations. The lack of genotype phenotype correlation for some genetic disorders, such as CF, also can limit the ability to accurately predict the course of the disease. Therefore, when molecular testing indicates that a patient or fetus has inherited a mutation, it is helpful to consult a geneticist or someone with expertise in the specific disorder to provide current information regarding the prognosis, as well as, the limitations and accuracy of testing.

APPLICATIONS IN OBSTETRICS AND GYNECOLOGY

Genetics is taking an increasingly prominent role in the practice of obstetrics and gynecology. Gene identification, characterization of disease-causing mutations, and advances in genetic technology have led to an increased number of available genetic tests, which may be used for the diagnosis of genetic disorders, carrier detection, and prenatal or preimplantation genetic diagnosis. Testing for a specific genetic disorder most often occurs in an obstetric setting based on either the family history or the couple's ethnicity. Genetic counseling should be offered to couples at risk so they can review the nature of the disorder, the inheritance pattern, their specific risk for being a carrier and for having a child with the disorder, the current availability of prenatal and postnatal testing as well the accuracy and limitations of testing, and their reproductive options. Most molecular genetic testing for disorders, such as Duchenne muscular dystrophy, fragile X syndrome, neurofibromatosis, and hemophilia, is performed when a couple is at high risk based on their family history. Initially, testing is performed to determine whether the parent is a carrier. If the parent is a carrier, prenatal testing by amniocentesis or chorionic villus sampling is possible. Some couples may consider preimplantation genetic diagnosis. Single gene disorders and chromosomal abnormalities, such as deletions and translocations, may be identified in an embryo conceived through in vitro fertilization by testing a single blastomere. Genetic testing for disorders prevalent in specific ethnic populations such as CF for Caucasians and Tay–Sachs and Canavan disease for individuals of Eastern European Jewish ancestry, is used to determine if an individual is a carrier. Prenatal molecular diagnostic testing is available for couples who are both carriers of sickle cell disease and thalassemia determined by hemoglobin electrophoresis. The genetic testing options in pregnancy are rapidly growing with the completion of the human genome project; however, a thorough family history is essential to identify a couple at risk.

Genetic testing during pregnancy may establish a diagnosis that may influence obstetric management. For example, PCR of amniotic fluid is used to determine the Rh status of the fetus to determine if the fetus is at risk for hemolytic disease of the newborn when the woman is Rh sensitized and the man is a heterozygous carrier of antigen D. The fetus at risk will need close surveillance during the pregnancy. A specific molecular diagnostic test may be considered when the finding of a fetal malformation by ultrasonography raises the suspicion of a genetic disorder. For example, mutation testing for CF in a fetus with echogenic bowel, fibroblast growth factor receptor 2 (FGFR2) for suspected Apert's syndrome (craniosynostosis), and 22q11.2 deletion testing when a conotruncal cardiac defect is detected. Identification of an etiology provides the physician and couple with a better understanding of the prognosis that influences not only the obstetric and neonatal care of the infant but also a couple's reproductive decisions. Furthermore, it establishes an accurate assessment of the recurrence risk for this family and their relatives.

Some of the genes responsible for the inherited forms of some types of cancer (such as breast, ovarian, and colon) have been identified. Risk assessment for relatives in these families may include genetic testing in addition to evaluating other risk factors, such as family history. In some families, breast and ovarian cancer is attributed to an inherited genetic mutation, *BRCA1* or *BRCA2*. The genes responsible for hereditary nonpolyposis colorectal cancer, juvenile polyposis, and familial adenomatosis polyposis, have been identified. It is likely that other genes that contribute to cancer will be identified in the future, which may be useful for cancer risk assessment and management.

Genetic screening and testing should be considered a component of an infertility evaluation. Preconceptional genetic screening and counseling can identify couples at risk for having offspring with a genetic disorder and provide them with information that enables them to make informed decisions regarding their reproductive options. Genetic causes of severe oligospermia and azoospermia include balanced translocations, Klinefelter's syndrome (47,XXY), and Y chromosome abnormalities and microdeletions. Cytogenetic studies and PCR-based Y chromosome deletion testing should be considered. Approximately two thirds of males with congenital bilateral absence of the vas deferens have at least one CF mutation. Men with congenital bilateral absence of the vas deferens should be offered CF carrier testing. Partners of carriers and individuals with CF should be tested to assess their risk for having a child with CF. This information may be useful for an infertile couple considering their reproductive options, such as testicular aspiration and biopsy with intracytoplasmic sperm injection, preimplantation genetic diagnosis with in vitro fertilization, donor gamete, adoption, and prenatal testing.

Summary

Human genetics and molecular testing is playing an increasingly important role in obstetric and gynecologic practice. It is essential that obstetricians and gynecologists are aware of the advances in our understanding of genetic disease and the fundamental principles of molecular testing and genetic screening as genetics is integrated into routine medical practice. In the future, elucidation of the genetic basis for reproductive disorders, common diseases, and cancer with improved high throughput technology for genetic testing will expand testing opportunities and influence treatment options and prevention strategies.

Reference

1. The human genome. Science 2001;291:1145–1434

Resources

Bell J. The new genetics in clinical practice. BMJ 1998;316: 618–620

Blackwood MA, Weber BL. BRCA1 and BRCA2: from molecular genetics to clinical medicine. J Clin Oncol 1998;16: 1969–1977

Brown PO, Botstein D. Exploring the new world of the genome with DNA microassays. Nat Genet 1999;21(suppl):33–37

Caskey CT. Medical genetics. JAMA 1997;277:1869–1870

Collins FS. Genetics: an explosion of knowledge is transforming clinical practice. Geriatrics 1999;54:41–47;quiz 48

Cooper DN, Schmidtke J. Diagnosis of human genetic disease using recombinant DNA. 4th ed. Hum Genet 1993;92:211–236

Davis JG. Predictive genetic tests: problems and pitfalls. Ann N Y Acad Sci 1997;833:42–46

Jameson JL. Principles of molecular medicine. Totowa, New Jersey: Humana Press, 1998

Korf B. Molecular diagnosis (1). N Engl J Med 1995;332: 1218–1220

Korf B. Molecular diagnosis (2). N Engl J Med 1995;332: 1499–1502

Makowski DR. The Human Genome Project and the clinician. J Fla Med Assoc 1996;83:307–314

Mark HF, Jenkins R, Miller WA. Current applications of molecular cytogenetic technologies. Ann Clin Lab Sci 1997;27: 47–56

Pyeritz RE. Family history and genetic risk factors: forward to the future. JAMA 1997;278:1284–1285

SOURCES OF ONLINE INFORMATION

Tutorial in Genetics (HHMI)
www.hhmi.org/GeneticTrail/

Online Mendelian Inheritance in Man
www3.ncbi.nlm.nih.gov/Omim/

MEDLINE
www.ncbi.nlm.nih.gov/PubMed/

GeneTests
www.genetests.org

Genome Database
www.gob.org

Biochemical testing information
biochemgen.ucsd.edu/wbgtests/dz.tst.htm

Alliance of Genetic Support Groups
medhlp.netusa.net/www/agsg.htm

National Human Genome Research
www.nhgri.nih.gov

Centers for Disease Control and Prevention
www.cdc.gov/genetics

Gene Clinics
www.geneclinics.org

GLOSSARY

Allele: One of two or more alternate forms of a gene.

Allele specific oligonucleotides: Synthetic oligonucleotide designed to hybridize to a specific sequence, and under the right conditions, to fail to hybridize to a related sequence. Allele specific oligonucleotides also are used as PCR primers in several methods similarly designed to distinguish between closely related alleles.

Autosomal Dominant: An allele located on an autosome (nonsex chromosome) that expresses itself phenotypically in the presence of the same or a different allele (ie, in a homozygous or heterozygous condition).

Autosomal Recessive: An allele located on an autosome that does not express itself phenotypically in the presence of a dominant allele (ie, in a heterozygous condition). It is only phenotypically expressed in a homozygous condition.

Chimera: An organism with tissues composed of two or more genetically distinct cell types.

Chromatin: An intranuclear and intrachromosomal complex made up of DNA, and histone and nonhistone proteins.

Co-Dominant: Alleles that are different from each other, but both are expressed in the phenotype.

Codon: A section of DNA (three nucleotide pairs in length) that codes for a single amino acid.

Comparative Genomic Hybridization: A cytogenetic method based on a combination of fluorescence microscopy and digital image analysis. Differentially labeled test DNA and normal reference DNA are hybridized simultaneously to normal chromosome spreads. Hybridization is detected with two different fluorochromes. Deletions, duplications, or amplifications are seen as changes in the ratio of the intensities of the two fluorochromes along the target chromosomes.

Complementary DNA (cDNA) Probe: A DNA sequence that is exactly complementary to mRNA, lacking introns and regulatory regions.

Contiguous Gene Deletion Syndrome: A syndrome caused by a deletion involving genes that are physically located together in a chromosome segment.

Constitutive Heterochromatin: Condensed genetically inactive chromatin located in the same regions of both homologous chromosomes.

DNA: A double-helical structure composed of two coils of nucleotide chains connected by nitrogen bases.

DNA Hybridization: A process whereby labeled nucleic acid molecules (oligonucleotide probe) bind to a DNA sequence on a target (Southern blot, metaphase chromosomes, or interphase nuclei) that is complementary to its own.

DNA Methylation: A process for control of tissue specific gene expression. Methylation "turns off" the regulatory region of a gene, thereby preventing DNA transcription.

Epigenetic: Non–DNA/RNA related process that affects genotype and phenotype (ie, methalization).

Exon: A region of a gene made up of DNA sequences that will be transcribed into mRNA.

Expressivity: The degree to which a genotype is expressed in the phenotype (range of phenotypic features).

Fluorescence in situ Hybridization (FISH): A procedure for detecting specific nucleic acid sequences in morphologically preserved chromosomes, cells, and tissue sections using fluorescent labeled oligonucleotide probes.

Gene: A unit of heredity responsible for the inheritance of a specific trait that occupies a fixed chromosomal site and corresponds to a sequence of nucleotides along a DNA molecule.

Genome: The entire complement of genetic material in a chromosome set.

Genomic Imprinting: The existence of parent-of-origin differences in the expression of certain genes.

Germline Mosaicism: Mosaicism that is confined to the gonad.

Hereditary Unstable DNA (Triplet Repeat Expansion): Gene containing a region of triplet codon repeats such as $(CGC)_n$. The number of triplet repeats can increase during meiosis. If the expansion of repeats reaches a critical number, the gene becomes methylated and is turned off, resulting in phenotypic abnormalities.

Heterochromatin: Chromatin that remains condensed throughout interphase. It contains DNA that is genetically inactive and replicates late in the S phase of the cell cycle. There are two types of heterochromatin: constitutive and facultative.

Hybridization (Dot Blot): A semiquantitative technique for evaluating the relative abundance of nucleic acid sequences in a mixture or the extent of similarity between homologous sequences.

Imprinting: The imposition of a stable behavior pattern in a young animal by exposure, during a particular period in its development, to one of a restricted set of stimuli.

Intron: A region of a gene, made up of noncoding DNA sequences that lies between exons.

Karyotype: The chromosome constitution of an individual.

Linkage: The association of genes on the same chromosome.

Methylation: (see DNA Methylation)

Mitochondrial Inheritance: Mitochondria are inherited exclusively from women. Because they contain DNA, mitochondrial inheritance allows transmission of genes directly from the woman to her offspring.

Mosaicism: The presence of two or more populations of cells with different characteristics within one tissue or organ.

Multifactorial Inheritance: Inheritance of traits that are determined by a combination of genetic and environmental factors.

Mutation: An alteration of DNA sequencing in a gene that results in a heritable change in protein structure or function that frequently has adverse effects.

> **Deletion:** A mutation that is generated by removal of a sequence of DNA, with the regions on either side being joined together.
>
> **Expansion** (see Hereditary Unstable DNA)
>
> **Frame-shift:** A mutation caused by deletions or insertions that are not a multiple of three base pairs. Results in a change in the reading frame in which triplet codons are translated into protein.
>
> **Insertion:** A mutation caused by the presence of an additional sequence of nucleotide pairs in DNA.
>
> **Inversion:** A mutation involving the removal of a DNA sequence, its rotation through 180 degrees, and its reinsertion in the same location.
>
> **Missense:** A mutation that alters a codon so that it encodes a different amino acid.

Northern Blot: A technique for transferring RNA from an electrophoresis gel to a nitrocellulose filter on which it can be hybridized to a complementary DNA (cDNA) probe.

Nucleotide: A component of a DNA or RNA molecule composed of a nitrogenous base, one deoxyribose or ribose sugar, and one phosphate group. In DNA, adenine specifically joins to thymine and guanine joins to cytosine. In RNA, uracil replaces thymine.

Oligonucleotide Primer: A short sequence of nucleotides that is necessary to hybridize to a DNA or RNA strand using the enzymes DNA polymerase or reverse transcriptase.

Penetrance: The ability of a mutant gene to be expressed in an individual who carries the gene.

Phenotype: Observable physical characteristics of an organism resulting from the expression of the genotype and its interaction with the environment.

Polygenic Inheritance: Inheritance of traits that are determined by the combined effects of many genes.

Polymerase Chain Reaction (PCR): A method for enzymatically amplifying a short sequence of DNA through repeated cycles of denaturation, binding with an oligonucleotide primer and extension of the primers by a DNA polymerase.

Polymorphisms: Minor differences that distinguish one individual from another.

Recombinant DNA: A new DNA sequence formed by the combination of two nonhomologous DNA molecules.

Restriction Endonuclease: An enzyme that recognizes and cleaves a specific DNA sequence (usually 4–10 nucleotide bases long).

Restriction Fragment Length Polymorphism: A polymorphic difference in DNA sequence between individuals that can be recognized by restriction endonucleases.

Southern Blot: A technique used to detect specific DNA sequences by separating restriction enzyme digested DNA fragments on an electrophoresis gel, transferring (blotting) these fragments from the gel onto a membrane or nitrocellulose filter, followed by hybridization with a labeled probe to a specific DNA sequence.

Spectral Karyotype: A molecular cytogenetic method in which all of the chromosomes in a metaphase spread are visualized in different colors (multicolor FISH).

Uniparental Disomy: Inheritance of two copies of part or all of a chromosome from one parent and no copy from the other parent.

Uniparental Heterodisomy: Inheritance of two homologous chromosomes from one parent.

Uniparental Isodisomy: Inheritance of two identical chromosomes from one parent.

Threshold Traits: Traits that are not manifested until a certain threshold of liability is exceeded.

Transcription: The process of RNA synthesis from a DNA template that is directed by RNA polymerase.

Triplet Repeat Expansion (see Hereditary Unstable DNA)

Trinucleotide Repeat Analysis (Repeats): Unstable DNA sequences found in several human genes. Normally the triplets are repeated in tandem 5–50 times. When the number rises above the normal range, mutant disease syndromes appear.

X-inactivation: A process by which one of the X chromosomes in each somatic cell of females is rendered inactive. This results in a balance in gene expression between the X chromosomal and autosomal genes, which is necessary because males have only one X chromosome.

X-linked: An allele for a trait or disorder that is located on the X chromosome. May be either dominant or recessive.

Western Blot: A technique, conceptually related to the Southern and Northern blot that is used to detect specific proteins.

ACOG Committee Opinion

Committee on Genetics

Number 189, October 1997

Advanced Paternal Age:

Risks to the Fetus

Advanced maternal age increases the risk of having a liveborn infant with autosomal trisomies 21, 18, or 13, or with the sex chromosome aneuploidies 47,XXY or 47,XXX. Genetic counseling traditionally has been offered when a woman will be 35 years of age or older as of her estimated delivery date. With increased paternal age, however, there does not appear to be an increased risk of chromosomal anomalies in offspring. Insufficient evidence exists to provide a specific cutoff level for assessing risk in association with paternal age.

Although advancing paternal age does affect pregnancy outcome, effects on genetic disease are less completely understood. There is general agreement that advancing paternal age predisposes the fetus to mutations in autosomal dominant diseases such as neurofibromatosis, achondroplasia, Apert syndrome, and Marfan syndrome. The increased risk rises exponentially, rather than linearly, with increasing paternal age. Increasing paternal age may be associated with spontaneous germline mutations in X-linked genes that are transmitted through carrier daughters to affected grandsons. This phenomenon has been called the "grandfather effect" and may occur with several X-linked disorders, including hemophilia A and Duchenne muscular dystrophy.

Although paternal age affects autosomal dominant diseases, the exact risk for any specific disorder is small. Most of the autosomal dominant diseases affect only 1 in 5,000–10,000 individuals, so even a doubling of risk constitutes a very low overall risk. It is the collective risk of autosomal dominant diseases that constitutes the increased risk, not the risk of a particular disorder.

Currently, it is not possible to screen prenatally for all autosomal dominant and X-linked diseases in the presence of advanced paternal age. Fetal ultrasonography may detect some autosomal dominant disorders, but this technique cannot be relied upon as a screening modality. Chromosomal analysis cannot be used to detect these disorders. Only genetic counseling on an individual basis is recommended for couples to address their specific concerns if advancing paternal age is an issue.

ISSN 1074-861X

The American College of Obstetricians and Gynecologists
409 12th Street, SW
PO Box 96920
Washington, DC 20090-6920

Bibliography

American College of Medical Genetics. Statement on guidance for genetic counseling in advanced paternal age. Bethesda, Maryland: ACMG, 1996

Ashton GC. Mismatches in genetic markers in a large family study. Am J Hum Genet 1980;32:601–613

de Michelena MI, Burstein E, Lama JR, Vasquez JC. Paternal age as a risk factor for Down syndrome. Am J Med Genet 1993;45:679–682

Friedman JM. Genetic disease in the offspring of older fathers. Obstet Gynecol 1981;57:745–749

Hook EB. A search for a paternal-age effect upon cases of 47, +21 in which the extra chromosome is of paternal origin. Am J Hum Genet 1984;36:413–421

McIntosh GC, Olshan AF, Baird PA. Paternal age and the risk of birth defects in offspring. Epidemiology 1995;6:282–288

Olshan AF, Anath CV, Savitz DA. Intrauterine growth retardation as an endpoint in mutation epidemiology: an evaluation based on paternal age. Mutat Res 1995;344:89–94

Olshan AF, Schnitzer PG, Baird PA. Paternal age and the risk of congenital heart defects. Teratology 1994;50:80–84

Risch N, Reich EW, Wishnick MM, McCarthy JG. Spontaneous mutation and parental age in humans. Am J Hum Genet 1987;41:218–248

ACOG Committee Opinion

Committee on Genetics

Number 239, August 2000 (Replaces No. 176, October 1996)

Breast–Ovarian Cancer Screening

This opinion was developed in consultation with Francis S. Collins, MD, PhD, Director of the National Human Genome Research Institute. This document reflects emerging clinical and scientific advances as of the date issued and is subject to change. The information should not be construed as dictating an exclusive course of treatment or procedure to be followed.

ISSN 1074-861X

The American College of Obstetricians and Gynecologists
409 12th Street, SW
PO Box 96920
Washington, DC 20090-6920

Based upon current knowledge, an estimated 5–7% of all breast and ovarian cancer is attributed to inherited mutations in two highly penetrant autosomal dominant susceptibility genes, *BRCA 1* and *BRCA 2*. In the general population, the gene frequency for *BRCA 1* and *BRCA 2* is low, occurring in approximately 1 in 800 individuals. Women who inherit either a *BRCA 1* or *BRCA 2* mutation have a 50–80% lifetime risk of breast cancer and an estimated 15–25% risk of developing ovarian cancer by age 70 years. *BRCA 1* appears to confer a higher risk of ovarian cancer than does *BRCA 2* (1, 2). *BRCA 2* is responsible for a much higher percentage of breast cancer cases in men. Mutations in *BRCA 1* and *BRCA 2* account for a substantial majority of inheritable breast cancers, while mutations in *p53*, H-*ras*, and the gene for ataxia–telangiectasia account for an additional small percentage. In the future, it is likely that other genes that contribute to the development of breast cancer will be discovered. Currently, reliance solely on genetic testing as a major predictor of breast and ovarian cancer is not supported by the science. An accurate evaluation of family history remains essential in assessing breast and ovarian cancer risk. Analysis has shown that multiple affected first- and second-degree relatives, both maternal and paternal, particularly with early onset disease, may significantly alter an individual's risk for breast and ovarian cancer (3).

BRCA 1 and *BRCA 2* are tumor suppressor genes. Women with a germline mutation in one copy of either gene have a decreased amount of the normal suppressor protein. Such individuals are at an increased risk of cancer if there is a loss of function in the normal copy of the gene. When this "second hit" occurs in a somatic cell (ie, breast cell), the result may be pathologic cell division.

Approximately 600 mutations in the *BRCA 1* gene and nearly 500 mutations of the *BRCA 2* gene have been found, of which 70–80% are thought to be disease producing. The precise biologic functions of *BRCA 1* and *BRCA 2* are still unclear.

The size of the *BRCA 1* gene, the widespread distribution of the mutations within the gene, the prevalence of different mutations in different populations, the technical problems in sequencing the entire gene, and the uncertain role of other gene pathways leading to breast–ovarian cancer in selected families make genetic testing for *BRCA 1* mutations an uncertain and incomplete science. In the future, it is possible that testing for the truncated protein product of the gene will be more practical for screening than DNA mutation analysis. Also contributing to the limitations of genetic testing for breast and ovarian cancer are the lack of understanding of the penetrance of the various mutations in diverse populations and the cost and benefit to the patient. For example, a single *BRCA 1* 185delAG mutation, previously identified in high-risk families, has been detected in approximately 1% of women of Eastern European Jewish descent. The true frequency of the mutation and implications of this finding are still uncertain, but there is a possibility that other *BRCA 1* mutations exist within the same population. For this reason, a negative test result for the *BRCA 1* 185delAG mutation alone would have little meaning in the presence of a strong family history of breast and ovarian cancer. Conversely, the interpretation of a positive test result for this mutation in the absence of a strong family history of cancer is unclear at present. Because identifying the precise mutations in a single affected relative makes looking for the same mutation in other family members easier, analysis usually begins with the DNA of an affected individual.

In selected families (multiple family members affected with breast or ovarian cancer, or a family in which a *BRCA* mutation has been discovered), *BRCA* testing may be useful. The failure to find a mutation in an individual, whose family has a known *BRCA* mutation, may reduce anxiety. The finding of a *BRCA* mutation in an individual with a strong family history for breast or ovarian cancer would allow the patient and physician to explore various management options. These might include more frequent surveillance, prophylactic surgery, such as mastectomy or oophorectomy, and trials of chemoprevention, such as oral contraceptives. Because of the problems previously described, testing of the general population is not recommended.

The Committee on Genetics of the American College of Obstetricians and Gynecologists believes that genetic testing for breast–ovarian cancer should be performed only with the individual's full informed consent. Currently, such testing continues to be best performed by investigators working under research protocols approved by an institutional review board. Individuals should be counseled before and after testing to ensure their understanding of the scope, implications, and limitations of the testing process. Counseling should include discussions of the uncertainties of applying genetic test results to the prevention and treatment of breast and ovarian cancer and the potential for genetic discrimination and loss of insurance coverage. The standard of care should emphasize genetic services, genetic information, and education and counseling, rather than the testing procedures alone. Although this document discusses DNA-based testing for inherited susceptibility to breast and ovarian cancer, the most important part of the screening process is obtaining and interpreting the family history. The National Cancer Institute Cancer Information Service (1-800-4-CANCER) can supply information about genetic services at cancer centers supported by the National Institutes of Health.

References

1. Burke W, Daly M, Garber J, Botkin J, Kahn MJ, Lynch P, et al. Recommendations for follow-up care of individuals with an inherited predisposition to cancer. II. BRCA1 and BRCA2. Cancer Genetics Studies Consortium. JAMA 1997;277:997–1003

2. Ford D, Easton DF, Bishop DT, Narod SA, Goldgar DE. Risks of cancer in BRCA1-mutation carriers. Breast Cancer Linage Consortium. Lancet 1994;343:692–695

3. Claus EB, Risch N, Thompson WD. Autosomal dominant inheritance early-onset breast cancer. Cancer 1994;73: 643–651

ACOG Committee Opinion

Committee on Genetics

Number 223, October 1999

First-Trimester Screening for Fetal Anomalies with Nuchal Translucency

ISSN 1074-861X

The American College of Obstetricians and Gynecologists
409 12th Street, SW
PO Box 96920
Washington, DC 20090-6920

Maternal serum screening in the second trimester of pregnancy is the current method of screening women at low risk for carrying fetuses with neural tube defects, certain chromosome abnormalities, and other select fetal malformations. This approach detects approximately 60% of Down syndrome cases in fetuses at a screen-positive rate of 5% (1). However, first-trimester screening for chromosome abnormalities offers many potential advantages over second-trimester screening. It helps reduce maternal anxiety at an earlier gestational age and allows the patient to take advantage of first-trimester prenatal diagnosis by chorionic villus sampling. If the fetus is found to be affected, the patient may elect to terminate the pregnancy. First-trimester pregnancy termination is associated with reduced maternal morbidity.

The ultrasonographic finding of nuchal translucency (an echo-free area at the back of the fetal neck) in the first trimester of pregnancy reportedly has been associated with fetal chromosome abnormalities (2–4). The prevalence of chromosome abnormalities is reported to vary from 30% to 86% in fetuses with increased nuchal translucency. Most of the early data on nuchal translucency screening involved high-risk women undergoing first-trimester prenatal diagnosis in referral centers for indications such as advanced maternal age or family history of a chromosome abnormality.

Studies involving low-risk women in a routine clinical practice setting have produced conflicting results (5–10). These differences appear to be attributable to interobserver and intraobserver variation in nuchal translucency measurements. In addition, there is no consensus on the definition of increased nuchal translucency (3, 4, 11). In most of the reports, the nuchal translucency measurements were taken from the sagittal section of the fetus usually used to obtain the crown–rump length (2–4). This appears to be the method of choice. However, some investigators have used a transverse suboccipitobregmatic view of the fetal head to obtain the measurement (11). When measuring nuchal translucency, care should be taken to distinguish nuchal skin from the amniotic membrane. Nuchal translucency values are crown–rump length-dependent (3, 4, 11, 12).

Nuchal Translucency Screening with Maternal Serum Screening Markers

Measurement of the free beta subunit of human chorionic gonadotropin and pregnancy-associated plasma protein-A in maternal serum appears promising as a method of screening for fetal chromosome abnormalities in the first trimester (13, 14). Similar to second-trimester screening, the Down syndrome detection rate with first-trimester biochemical screening is approximately 60% with a 5% screen-positive rate (14). Ongoing research indicates that combining first-trimester maternal serum screening markers with nuchal translucency screening may allow up to an 80–90% detection rate for Down syndrome (15, 16). These preliminary data remain controversial.

Using Nuchal Translucency to Screen for Fetal Cardiac Anomalies

Prenatal detection of fetal cardiac abnormalities currently is performed during second-trimester ultrasound examination. Of fetuses with chromosome abnormalities, 50–90% have major anomalies of the heart and great vessels. It is possible that the lymphedema seen in nuchal translucency is associated with fetal cardiac abnormalities (17). It also is possible that nuchal translucency in fetuses without chromosome abnormalities is cardiogenic in nature. In fetuses with normal chromosomes and nuchal translucency, it appears that the prevalence of major cardiac abnormalities increases with nuchal translucency size (17).

Recommendations

- First-trimester screening for fetal chromosome, cardiac, and other abnormalities using the nuchal translucency marker alone or in combination with serum markers appears promising but remains investigational.
- The technique for measuring nuchal translucency and the criteria for defining increased nuchal translucency must be standardized.
- Until further studies confirm the efficacy of first-trimester nuchal translucency screening, with or without serum markers, this modality is not recommended for routine clinical use.

References

1. Haddow JE, Palomaki GE, Knight GJ, Williams J, Pulkkinen A, Canick JA, et al. Prenatal screening for Down's syndrome with use of maternal serum markers. N Engl J Med 1992;327:588–593
2. Bronshtein M, Rottem S, Yoffe N, Blumenfeld Z. First-trimester and early second-trimester diagnosis of nuchal cystic hygroma by transvaginal sonography: diverse prognosis of the septated from the nonseptated lesion. Am J Obstet Gynecol 1989;161:78–82
3. Nicolaides KH, Azar G, Byrne D, Mansur C, Marks K. Fetal nuchal translucency: ultrasound screening for chromosomal defects in first trimester of pregnancy. BMJ 1992; 304:867–869
4. Nicolaides KH, Brizot ML, Snijders RJ. Fetal nuchal translucency: ultrasound screening for fetal trisomy in the first trimester of pregnancy. Br J Obstet Gynaecol 1994; 101:782–786
5. Pajkrt E, de Graaf IM, Mol BW, van Lith JM, Bleker OP, Bilardo CM. Weekly nuchal translucency measurements in normal fetuses. Obstet Gynecol 1998;91:208–211
6. Kornman LH, Morssink LP, Beekhius JR, De Wolf BT, Heringa MP, Mantingh A. Nuchal translucency cannot be used as a screening test for chromosomal abnormalities in the first trimester of pregnancy in a routine ultrasound practice. Prenat Diagn 1996;16:797–805
7. Roberts LJ, Bewley S, Mackinson AM, Rodeck CH. First trimester fetal nuchal translucency: problems with screening the general population. 1. Br J Obstet Gynaecol 1995; 102:381–385
8. Bewley S, Roberts LJ, Mackinson AM, Rodeck CH. First trimester fetal nuchal translucency: problems with screening the general population. 2. Br J Obstet Gynaecol 1995; 102:386–388
9. Hafner E, Schuchter K, Philipp K. Screening for chromosomal abnormalities in an unselected population by fetal nuchal translucency. Ultrasound Obstet Gynecol 1995;6: 330–333
10. Hafner E, Schuchter K, Liebhart E, Philipp K. Results of routine fetal nuchal translucency measurement at weeks 10–13 in 4233 unselected pregnant women. Prenat Diagn 1998;18:29–34
11. Comas C, Martinez JM, Ojuel J, Casals E, Puerto B, Borell A, et al. First-trimester nuchal edema as a marker of aneuploidy. Ultrasound Obstet Gynecol 1995;5:26–29
12. Schuchter K, Wald N, Hackshaw AK, Hafner E, Liebhart E. The distribution of nuchal translucency at 10-13 weeks of pregnancy. Prenat Diagn 1998;18:281–286
13. Macri JN, Spencer K, Aitken D, Garver K, Buchanan PD, Muller F, et al. First-trimester free beta (hCG) screening for Down syndrome. Prenat Diagn 1993;13:557–562
14. Krantz DA, Larsen JW, Buchanan PD, Macri JN. First-trimester Down syndrome screening: free beta-human chorionic gonadotropin and pregnancy-associated plasma protein A. Am J Obstet Gynecol 1996;174:612–616
15. Orlandi F, Damiani G, Hallahan TW, Krantz DA, Macri JN. First-trimester screening for fetal aneuploidy: biochemistry and nuchal translucency. Ultrasound Obstet Gynecol 1997;10:381–386
16. Spencer K, Noble P, Snijders RJ, Nicolaides KH. First-trimester urine free beta hCG, beta core, and total oestriol in pregnancies affected by Down's syndrome: implications for first-trimester screening with nuchal translucency and serum free beta hCG. Prenat Diagn 1997;17:525–538
17. Hyett JA, Perdu M, Sharland GK, Snijders RS, Nicolaides KH. Increased nuchal translucency at 10–14 weeks of gestation as a marker for major cardiac defects. Ultrasound Obstet Gynecol 1997;10:242–246

ACOG Committee Opinion

Committee on Genetics

Number 161, October 1995

Fragile X Syndrome

Fragile X syndrome is the most common inherited form of mental retardation, affecting about 1 in 1,500 males and 1 in 2,500 females from a variety of ethnic backgrounds. Mental retardation ranges from borderline to severe, although most patients have moderate degrees of mental retardation. Other associated phenotypic abnormalities include autistic behaviors, macroorchidism in adult males, characteristic narrow face with a large jaw, and speech and language problems. The abnormal facial features are subtle and become more noticeable with age, making phenotypic diagnosis difficult, especially in the newborn.

Standard metaphase chromosomal analysis does not consistently demonstrate the cytogenetic abnormality in patients with fragile X syndrome. Using specific culture conditions (folate deprivation), the demonstration of a fragile site on the long (q) arm of the human X chromosome (Xq27-28) was identified in males and some females with fragile X syndrome. The syndrome was originally thought to be transmitted in a classic X-linked recessive fashion; however, the inheritance of fragile X syndrome has proven to be much more complex. Females may be affected. Nearly all males with fragile X and most carrier females who have mental retardation show the fragile site. However, about 20% of males with the mutant gene do not have mental retardation and do not demonstrate cytogenetic evidence of the fragile site. These men are referred to as transmitting males. Two thirds of carrier females are mentally normal, and only one third of these demonstrate cytogenetic findings. These variations in the expression of the fragile site complicate cytogenetic diagnosis, particularly prenatal diagnosis. Molecular diagnostic techniques have now replaced cytogenetic analysis as the diagnostic procedure of choice for the fragile X syndrome.

The molecular cloning of the fragile X mental retardation-1 gene (*FMR*-1) has helped to clarify the molecular basis of the fragile X syndrome. Nearly all of the mutations in the gene involve expansion of a triplet repeat consisting of the bases cytosine–guanine–guanine. This pattern appears to correlate with the fragile site detected by cytogenetic techniques. The number of repeats varies in unaffected individuals (Table 1). A patient with 50–200 repeats is phenotypically normal and is said to have a premutation. When greater than 200 repeats are present, the patient has a full mutation that results in phenotypic fragile X syndrome. The *FMR-1* gene nearly always becomes methylated and inactivated in these patients. The number of repeats and the status of gene methylation are determined by using DNA-based mol-

ISSN 1074-861X

The American College of Obstetricians and Gynecologists
409 12th Street, SW
Washington, DC 20024-2188

Table 1. Mutation in the Fragile X Mental Retardation-1 Gene

Status of Individual	Number of Triplet Repeats (Cytosine–Guanine–Guanine)
Unaffected	6–49
Premutation	50–200
Full mutation	>200

ecular tests (ie, Southern blot analysis and polymerase chain reaction). Chorionic villus sampling may not be reliable for diagnosis because of different methylation patterns in the trophoblast as compared with the fetus. Although reliable for determining the number of triplet repeats, chorionic villus sampling may not adequately determine the methylation status of the *FMR-1* gene.

Transmission of a disease-producing mutation to a fetus depends upon the sex of the parent and the number of cytosine–guanine–guanine repeats present in the parental gene. Parents at risk for transmission of the disease are those who have either the premutation or the full DNA mutation. When a female carries the premutation and the length of the repeat exceeds 90, premutation genes are much more likely to expand and to result in the birth of an affected child. Males may transmit the premutation gene to their children, but expansion to a full mutation has not been described in the offspring of a male having the premutation gene. Empirically determined risks are available for the purposes of genetic counseling. An antibody-based test using peripheral blood is currently under investigation as a rapid approach to the screening of mentally retarded individuals and neonates for fragile X syndrome (1).

The Committee recommends the following regarding testing for fragile X syndrome:

1. DNA-based molecular analysis is the preferred method of diagnosis for fragile X syndrome and its premutations. Cytogenetic analysis should not be used for the definitive diagnosis of fragile X syndrome.
2. Testing for fragile X syndrome should be considered in any child with developmental delay of uncertain etiology or any individual with mental retardation of uncertain etiology. If there is no DNA evidence for the fragile X syndrome in an individual with mental retardation, standard chromosome analysis may also be considered in order to exclude chromosomal causes of mental retardation such as autosomal trisomies, deletions, duplications, or unbalanced translocations.
3. Patients with a family history of mental retardation or a history of fragile X mental retardation should undergo genetic evaluation to assess their risk for having an affected child.
4. Prenatal testing for fragile X syndrome by amniocentesis should be offered to known carriers of the fragile X premutation or mutation.

References

1. Willemsen R, Mohkamsing S, De Vries B, Devys D, van den Ouweland A, Mandel JL, et al. Rapid antibody test for fragile X syndrome. Lancet 1995;345:1147–1148
2. Warren ST, Nelson DL. Advances in molecular analysis of fragile X syndrome. JAMA 1994;271:536–542
3. Nussbaum RL, Ledbetter DH. The fragile X syndrome. In: Scriver CR, Beaudet AL, Sly WS, Valle D, eds. The metabolic basis of inherited disease. 6th ed. Vol I. New York: McGraw-Hill Inc, 1989:327–341
4. The American College of Medical Genetics policy statement. Fragile X syndrome: diagnostic and carrier testing. Bethesda, Maryland: Working Group of the Genetic Screening Subcommittee of the Clinical Practice Committee, ACMG, July 22, 1994, pages 1–4

ACOG

Committee on Genetics

Committee Opinion

Number 257, May 2001 *(Replaces No. 178, November 1996)*

Genetic Evaluation of Stillbirths and Neonatal Deaths

In the burgeoning field of genetics, a complete evaluation of stillbirths and neonatal deaths yields more information than in the past. Autopsy findings supplemented by genetic studies may provide important information (1). This information may explain the cause of death, direct further investigation of the family, and be particularly valuable in counseling parents about recurrence risks in future pregnancies.

Parental Consent

It is important to obtain parental consent; however, grief stricken parents may be reticent to consent to autopsy examination. They may view it as a violation of the sanctity of the dead body or as serving the physician's interests or curiosity. Even though bereaved parents may not want the information initially, care providers should strongly emphasize that results of the evaluation may be useful to the patient and her family in planning future pregnancies. If still reluctant to consent to a full autopsy, the family should be informed of the value of less invasive methods of evaluation, including photographs, X-rays, and sampling of tissues, such as blood or skin. These methods may help to identify a syndrome or chromosomal abnormality even without full autopsy data. Congenital anomalies are a significant cause of fetal death; 15–20% of stillbirths have a major malformation. Approximately 8% of stillbirths have chromosomal abnormalities and about 20% have dysmorphic features or skeletal abnormalities (2, 3). Malformations often are present in patterns that permit classification into a particular syndrome. Syndrome identification may delineate etiologic and pathogenetic factors that could have predictive significance for recurrence risk and the risk of other associated anomalies (4). Also, it is important to note that in addition to genetic causes, some fetal and neonatal deaths are caused by obstetric or medical complications for which preventive measures may be available.

This document reflects emerging clinical and scientific advances as of the date issued and is subject to change. The information should not be construed as dictating an exclusive course of treatment or procedure to be followed

ISSN 1074-861X

The American College of Obstetricians and Gynecologists
409 12th Street, SW
PO Box 96920
Washington, DC 20090-6920

Management

After a stillbirth or neonatal death, proper management includes a careful perinatal and family history, a physical examination of the fetus or infant (with documentation by description and photography, if possible), and indicated laboratory studies (see box). To ascertain the etiology and provide appropriate counseling to the family, clinical–pathologic correlation is best accomplished by a team comprising obstetricians, pediatricians, neonatologists, pathologists, and geneticists.

History

When stillbirth or neonatal death occurs, the obstetric history including exposures (eg, medications, viral infections), and family history, including a three-generation pedigree if possible, should be reviewed. Any pertinent information in the maternal or paternal pedigree should be documented and investigated further. Relevant original medical records and documentation should be obtained whenever possible. The gestational age by last menstrual period, maternal examinations, laboratory data, and ultrasonograms should be recorded for correlation with the physical examination of the neonate. Possible nongenetic causes also should be considered.

Examination of the Stillbirth

The general examination of the stillborn infant should be done promptly, noting any dysmorphic features and obtaining body measurements, including crown–rump, crown–heel, and foot lengths, as well as weight (5–8). Foot length is especially useful before 23 weeks of gestation. These measurements help estimate gestational age and evaluate intrauterine growth. Further documentation by frontal and profile photographs, with close-ups of specific abnormalities, is valuable for subsequent review and consultations. Even if parents have declined an autopsy, a description of any obvious abnormalities of the stillbirth should be included in the medical record.

X-rays, examination of the placenta, and autopsy should be considered. This is especially true when dysmorphic features, inconsistent growth measurements, anomalies, hydrops, or growth restriction is present. Whole body X-ray with anterior–posterior and lateral views may reveal an unrecognized skeletal abnormality or further define a grossly apparent deformity. If possible, the infant should be positioned with extremities extended and the epiphyses viewed.

When a full autopsy is performed, it should follow the guidelines for perinatal autopsy published by the College of American Pathologists (www.cap.org) or other standard references (9, 10). The pathologist should be aware of the clinical history and suspected genetic diagnoses so that samples for cytogenetic, metabolic, and molecular studies may be taken.

Management of Stillbirth or Fetal Death*

- Obtain informed consent from parents for autopsy
- Obtain perinatal and family history
- Perform physical examination of fetus and describe findings
- Photograph fetus
- Perform whole body X-rays of fetus
- Perform autopsy of fetus
- Perform gross and microscopic examination of placenta
- Perform cytogenetic studies
- Perform biochemical, molecular genetic, or infectious disease studies as indicated

*If these services are not available at your hospital, consider sending to a regional hospital center or contact your state board of pathology.

Examination of the Placenta

Gross and microscopic examination of the placenta, membranes, and umbilical cord may corroborate autopsy findings or explain apparent fetal deformity. Gross evaluation of the umbilical cord and blood vessels, membranes for amniotic bands and other anomalies, and placenta for size and condition should be performed. Histologic study of placental samples also should be performed (11, 12).

Laboratory Studies

Samples of amniotic fluid, umbilical cord blood, or amnion may be obtained for chromosomal and any other relevant studies. Analysis of bile, vitreous humor, urine, and fetal tissue may be helpful if umbilical cord blood is unobtainable (13, 14). Guidelines for the procurement of samples for chromosomal and genetic studies are outlined in the box on the following page.

Chromosomal analysis of amniotic fluid or chorionic villi ideally should be offered as soon as a fetal death is recognized. Although this information can be obtained at the time of delivery, the likelihood of obtaining a karyotype is decreased if there is a long interval between fetal death and delivery. This is

Guidelines for the Procurement of Samples for Chromosomal and Genetic Studies

- Obtain consent to take skin, eye, body fluids, and other tissue samples (separate from autopsy consent).
- For cytogenetic and molecular genetic studies, the following samples are acceptable:
  —Umbilical cord blood (3 mL)
  —Skin with attached dermis (1 cm^2)
  —Fascia from thigh, inguinal region, or Achilles tendon (1 cm) especially when maceration of the skin is present; and
  —Kidney, skeletal, muscle, liver, lung, and gonads, if indicated.
- Samples should be obtained using sterile techniques as soon as possible.
- Umbilical cord blood should be placed into sterile tube with heparin.
- Tissue samples should be placed in appropriate sterile medium obtained from cytogenetic laboratory or in normal saline if medium is not available. Do not use fixative solutions (eg, formaldehyde).
- Samples should be kept at room temperature.
- Freeze a 1 cm tissue sample.

especially true when dysmorphic features, inconsistent growth measurements, anomalies, hydrops, or growth restriction are present, or when a parent carries a balanced chromosomal rearrangement (eg, translocation or inversion) or has a mosaic karyotype. Based on the history, examination of the fetus, radiographic studies, and autopsy findings, specific molecular or biochemical tests may be indicated. For example, fluorescence in situ hybridization studies used to identify a deletion of chromosome 22q11.2 should be considered when a conotruncal cardiac defect (eg, interrupted aortic arch, truncus arteriosus) is detected (15).

Counseling

The results of the autopsy, placental examination, laboratory tests, and cytogenetic studies should be communicated to the involved clinicians and to the family of the deceased infant in a timely manner. Further, the family should be counseled promptly after a consensus is reached. Counseling before the evaluation is complete or before different opinions of the various caregivers have been resolved may increase feelings of guilt or anger in parents who have experienced a perinatal death. When there is an abnormal child or a genetic defect, these feelings often are magnified. Specific testing of the parents may be offered. The results of the tests are important even when no specific diagnosis is identified (16). A list of diagnoses excluded may be useful in counseling the parents. Whether or not there is a specific diagnosis, compassionate counseling of the parents and sensitivity to their needs are required.

References

1. Saller DN Jr, Lesser KB, Harrel U, Rogers BB, Oyer CE. The clinical utility of the perinatal autopsy. JAMA 1995; 273:663–665
2. Pauli RM, Reiser CA. Wisconsin Stillbirth Service Program: II. Analysis of diagnoses and diagnostic categories in the first 1,000 referrals. Am J Med Genet 1994; 50:135–153
3. Pauli RM, Reiser CA, Lebovitz RM, Kirkpatrick SJ. Wisconsin Stillbirth Service Program: I. Establishment and assessment of a community-based program for etiologic investigation of intrauterine deaths. Am J Med Genet 1994;50:116–134
4. Leppig KA, Werler MM, Cann CI, Cook CA, Holmes LB. Predictive value of minor anomalies. I. Association with major malformations. J Pediatr 1987;110:531–537
5. Reed GB, Claireaux AE, Cockburn F, eds. Diseases of the fetus and newborn: pathology, imaging, genetics, and management. 2nd ed. London: Chapman and Hall Medical, 1995
6. Stocker JT, Dehner LP. Pediatric pathology. Philadelphia: Lippincott, 1992
7. Naeye RL. Disorders of the placenta, fetus, and neonate: diagnosis and clinical significance. St Louis: Mosby-Year Book, Inc, 1992
8. Shepard TH, Shi M, Fellingham GW, Fujinaga M, FitzSimmons JM, Fantel AG, et al. Organ weight standards for human fetuses. Pediatr Pathol 1988;8:513–524
9. Valdes-Dapena MA, Huff DS. Perinatal autopsy manual. Collingdale, Pennsylvania: Diane Publishing, 1993
10. Bove KE. Practice guidelines for autopsy pathology: the perinatal and pediatric autopsy. Autopsy Committee of the College of American Pathologists. Arch Pathol Lab Med 1997;121:368–376
11. Benirschke K, Kaufman P. Pathology of the human placenta. 4th ed. New York: Springer-Verlag, 2000
12. Genest DR. Estimating the time of death in stillborn fetuses: II. Histologic evaluation of the placenta; a study of 71 stillborns. Obstet Gynecol 1992;80:585–592
13. Emery JL, Howat AJ, Variend S, Vawter GF. Investigation of inborn errors of metabolism in unexpected infant deaths. Lancet 1988;2:29–31
14. Rashed MS, Ozand PT, Bennett MJ, Barnard JJ, Govindaraju DR, Rinaldo P. Inborn errors of metabolism diagnosed in sudden death cases by acylcarnitine analysis of postmortem bile. Clin Chem 1995;41:1109–1114
15. Goldmuntz E, Clark BJ, Mitchell LE, Jawad AF, Reed L, McDonald-McGinn D, et al. Frequency of 22q11 deletions in patients with conotruncal defects. J Am Coll Cardiol 1998;32:492–498
16. Rushton DI. Prognostic role of the perinatal postmortem. Br J Hosp Med 1994;52:450–454

ACOG

Committee on Genetics

Committee Opinion

Number 238, July 2000 *(Replaces No. 168, February 1996)*

Genetic Screening for Hemoglobinopathies

Over the past several years, genetics research has advanced our knowledge of disease-causing mutations in the hemoglobin genes and developed tests for their precise identification. These tests can identify couples at risk for offspring with hemoglobinopathies and provide them with information to make a decision about whether to have prenatal testing. Counseling couples at increased risk for hemoglobinopathies requires a knowledge of genotype and phenotype. The ever-widening ethnic and geographic distribution of human hemoglobinopathies has made the identification of individuals at increased risk by ethnic or racial origin less reliable. Obstetrician–gynecologists who offer genetic risk assessment need to be aware of risk factors and new developments in the ability to detect mutations in carriers and identify affected fetuses.

Initiation of screening for hemoglobinopathies depends on the patient's ethnic background, medical history, family history, and red blood cell indices and on the goals of testing. In many states, screening infants for hemoglobinopathies is routine. As a result, in the future couples may know their hemoglobin genotypes when they visit an obstetrician–gynecologist. Screening of all couples of reproductive age is not recommended; however, the obstetrician–gynecologist should try to identify couples at increased risk for having offspring with a form of thalassemia or sickle cell disease. Historically, high-risk groups include people of African-American, Southeast Asian, or Mediterranean ancestry. Ethnic groups considered to be at low risk for these disorders are northern European, Japanese, Inuit (Eskimo), Native American, and individuals of Mexican and Korean descent.

A combination of laboratory tests may be necessary to provide the information required for genetic counseling of patients who are carriers of α-thalassemia, β-thalassemia, or sickle cell anemia (Fig. 1). Patients of Southeast Asian descent are at an increased risk for α-thalassemia, and patients of Mediterranean descent are at an increased risk for β-thalassemia. To ensure accurate hemoglobin identification, which is needed for genetic counseling, electrophoresis is the appropriate initial laboratory test for individuals determined to be at risk for a hemoglobin disorder. Several tests, including solubility testing such as a test for the presence of hemoglobin S (Sickledex), isoelectric focusing, and high-performance liquid chromatography (HPLC), have been used for primary screening. Solubility tests are

This document reflects emerging clinical and scientific advances as of the date issued and is subject to change. The information should not be construed as dictating an exclusive course of treatment or procedure to be followed.

ISSN 1074-861X

The American College of Obstetricians and Gynecologists
409 12th Street, SW
PO Box 96920
Washington, DC 20090-6920

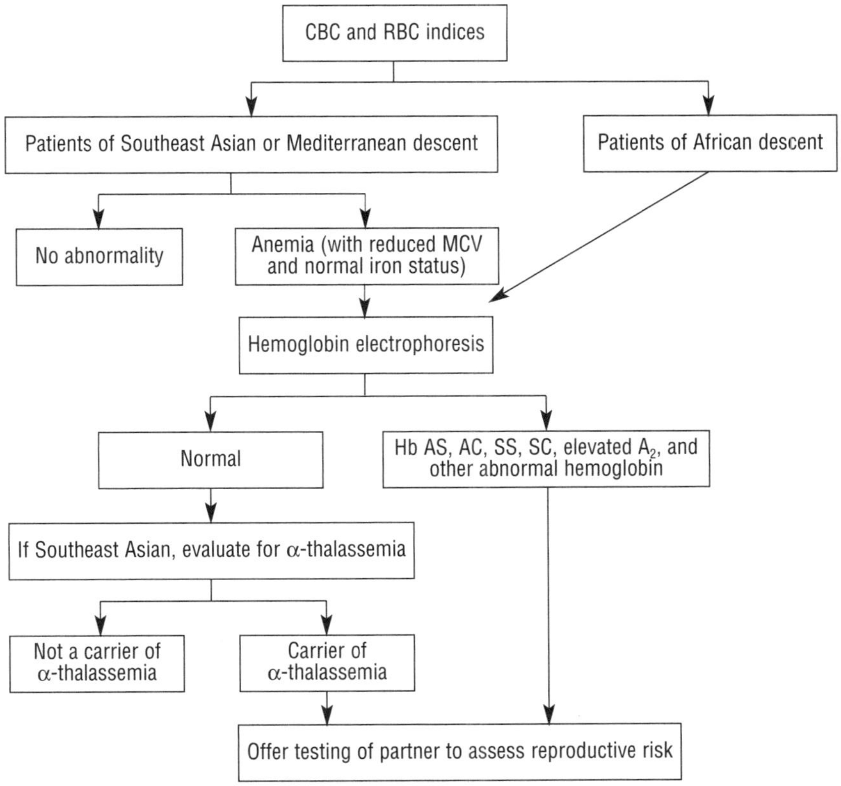

Fig. 1. Specialized antepartum evaluation for hematologic assessment of patients of African, Southeast Asian, or Mediterranean descent. Patients of Southeast Asian or Mediterranean descent should undergo electrophoresis if their blood test results reveal anemia. Abbreviations: CBC = complete blood count; RBC = red blood cell; MCV = mean corpuscular volume; Hb = hemoglobin.

inadequate because they fail to identify important transmissible hemoglobin gene abnormalities affecting fetal outcome. Solubility test results may be negative for individuals with an abnormal hemoglobin gene (eg, Hb C trait, β-thalassemia trait, Hb E trait, Hb B trait, Hb D trait). Many individuals with these genotypes are asymptomatic, but if their partners have sickle cell trait or other hemoglobinopathies, they may produce children with more serious hemoglobinopathies, such as Hb S/β-thalassemia and Hb SC disease. Solubility testing may be valuable, however, for rapidly screening for sickling when this information is critical for immediate patient care.

Determination of mean corpuscular volume (MCV) is recommended for patients who are at increased risk for α- or β-thalassemia. Patients who have a low MCV (<80 μ^3) may have one of the thalassemia traits and are candidates for hemoglobin electrophoresis. β-Thalassemia is associated with elevated fetal hemoglobin and elevated hemoglobin A_2 levels (>3.5%). Neither hemoglobin electrophoresis nor solubility testing will identify individuals with α-thalassemia or α-thalassemia trait; this condition can be identified only by molecular genetic testing. If the MCV is below normal, iron deficiency anemia has been excluded, and the hemoglobin electrophoresis is not consistent with β-thalassemia trait (ie, there is no elevation of hemoglobin A_2 or fetal hemoglobin), then DNA-based testing should be used to detect α-globin gene deletions characteristic of α-thalassemia. If both partners are identified as carriers of a gene for abnormal hemoglobins, counseling for DNA-based prenatal diagnostic testing should be offered.

References

1. Scriver CR, Beaudet AL, Sly WS, Valle D, eds. The metabolic and molecular basis of inherited disease. 7th ed. New York: McGraw-Hill, 1995
2. Guy G, Coady DJ, Jansen V, Snyder J, Zinberg S. alpha-Thalassemia hydrops fetalis: clinical and ultrasonographic considerations. Am J Obstet Gynecol 1985;153:500–504
3. Baysal E, Huisman TH. Detection of common deletional alpha-thalassemia-2 determinants by PCR. Am J Hematol 1994;46:208–213
4. Rimoin DL, Connor JM, Pyeritz RE, eds. Emery and Rimoin's principles and practice of medical genetics. 3rd ed. New York: Churchill Livingstone, 1997

ACOG

Committee on Genetics

Committee Opinion

Number 192, October 1997

Genetic Screening of Gamete Donors

When the risk to offspring is high and when prenatal diagnosis is not available or is not an acceptable alternative, the use of donor gametes is an option for couples with genetic risk factors. This is especially true if one member of the couple has a disabling autosomal dominant disorder or the couple already has a child with an autosomal recessive disorder for which prenatal diagnosis is not yet available. Even when prenatal diagnosis is available, some at-risk couples prefer gamete donation to therapeutic abortion. For others with genetic disorders that render them agonadal and infertile, gamete donation is an alternative to adoption that offers a biologic connection to the mother and control over the prenatal environment. In all such cases, gamete donation is one of the alternatives available through genetic counseling and assisted reproduction. When gamete donation is used, the Committee on Genetics recommends the clinical and genetic evaluation of all donors to avoid the transmission of heritable genetic disorders. There are other considerations when selecting a gamete donor, such as screening for infectious diseases; however, these will not be addressed in this Committee Opinion, which is limited to genetic evaluation.

Each physician should pay close attention to the number of times that a given individual in a population is used as a gamete donor. Otherwise, the rate of consanguinity might exceed that observed in the general population, and the incidence of recessive disorders might be increased. For example, if a given gamete donor is the carrier of a rare recessive mutation, excessive use of that donor might generate a cluster of similar carriers in a given locality. Over a 20- to 30-year period, this donor might generate more offspring who are homozygous for this rare autosomal recessive disorder than would otherwise have been the case. It is difficult to provide a precise number of times that a given donor can be used because one must take into consideration the population base from which the donor is selected and the catchment area that is served by the gamete donation facility. For example, to avoid inadvertent consanguinity equal to or greater than first-cousin marriages in a population of 800,000, assuming assorted mating, a single sperm donor should not be used to achieve more than 25 pregnancies (1, 2).

The most important part of the screening process is obtaining and interpreting the family history of the gamete donor in conjunction with the physical examination. A genetic questionnaire can be used as an adjunct to obtain this information. The emphasis should be on genetic information (ie, education and counseling) rather than testing procedures alone. This general

ISSN 1074-861X

The American College of Obstetricians and Gynecologists
409 12th Street, SW
PO Box 96920
Washington, DC 20090-6920

approach, coupled with selected testing, will help to reduce the risk of genetic diseases in this unique population of offspring.

Gamete Donors (General)

Regardless of the donor's sex, it is important to screen the donor's three-generation pedigree for any genetic disorders, perform a physical examination, and determine the donor's ethnic background. Genetic diseases in the following categories are especially important:

- Autosomal or X-linked disease with age of onset extending beyond the age of the donor (eg, Huntington's disease)
- Autosomal dominant disease with reduced penetrance or variable expressivity (eg, Marfan syndrome, neurofibromatosis)
- Autosomal recessive disease, especially if the disease has a high frequency in the population (eg, cystic fibrosis, Tay–Sachs disease)

Screening Tests

The D (Rho[D]) type of all gamete donors should be known. To minimize the small but unavoidable risk to D-negative women, this should include testing for D^u.

In addition to D typing, one should screen donors to determine their risk, on the basis of family history and ethnic background, of having offspring with the hemoglobinopathies, Tay–Sachs disease, and fragile X syndrome. However, universal screening for hemoglobinopathies is not recommended. Donors who are at increased risk for having offspring with the thalassemias should be screened initially with red-cell indices followed by hemoglobin electrophoresis. Individuals with a normal hemoglobin electrophoresis who are considered to be at risk for alpha-thalassemia require DNA analysis for precise genotyping. Patients at risk for having offspring with sickle cell disease should be screened with hemoglobin electrophoresis (3).

Donors who are of Ashkenazi Jewish, French-Canadian, or Cajun descent should be screened for Tay–Sachs carrier status. Screening of gamete donors for Tay–Sachs disease can be performed easily and rapidly using human serum.

Cystic fibrosis testing is controversial. Some have suggested that caucasian donors should be screened for cystic fibrosis because of its high carrier frequency of 1 in 25. However, general population screening of caucasians for cystic fibrosis currently is not being recommended and therefore cannot be recommended routinely for gamete donors at this time. Nevertheless, the opportunity for testing of the potential donor for cystic fibrosis may be offered as an option to the recipient of the donated gamete.

Donor Screening

A positive history in the donor or the donor's first-degree relatives (ie, parent, sibling, or offspring) of repetitive miscarriages should prompt a chromosomal analysis of the donor, regardless of the number of normal or abnormal liveborns or stillborns. Individuals who have a known balanced chromosomal rearrangement or who have previously had offspring with a chromosomal abnormality should be excluded as gamete donors.

To decrease the risk of aneuploid offspring, it is prudent to limit oocyte donors to women who are less than 35 years of age. The increased frequency of de novo mutations in sperm from older men suggests that sperm from younger men is preferable. To avoid consanguinity in gamete donation programs, the oocyte donor and the sperm donor should not be genetically related.

Embryo Recipient

Embryo recipients should be screened for antibodies against red-cell surface antigens to avoid isoimmune hemolytic disease of the fetus and newborn. Other assessments of the embryo recipient with respect to maternal health and susceptibility to disease (ie, rubella antibody titer, blood chemistries) are advisable as well.

The embryo recipient should undergo careful physical assessment to detect obstetric risk factors. This is especially critical when the indication for gamete donation is a genetic disorder in the embryo recipient that puts her at high risk (eg, gonadal dysgenesis, Marfan syndrome). In some of these genetic disorders, the embryo recipient has functional ovaries; in others, the embryo recipient is agonadal. In the former situation, the donor gamete is being used to reduce the risk of a genetically abnormal child; in the latter situation, a donor egg is essential for successful reproduction. Extrinsic, nongenetic factors that might pose a risk to the fetus or to the continuation of the pregnancy (eg, rubella antibody, uterine abnormalities) should be assessed continually. To reduce the incidence of neural tube defects, embryo recipients should receive 400 μg of folic acid per day starting 6–8 weeks prior to embryo transfer and continuing until the end of the first trimester of pregnancy.

General

Apart from a specific genetic disorder, certain gamete donors and donor–recipient combinations have cumulative or polygenic risk factors that currently cannot be easily quantitated or specified. Attempts to prevent genetic defects in gamete donors always will be imperfect, as they are in nonassisted reproduction. Due to limitations in current knowledge and technology, genetic heterogeneity, and unanticipated de novo germline mutations, unforeseen and unanticipated abnormalities cannot be prevented, despite the physician's best efforts.

References

1. deBoer A, Oosterwijk JC, Ritgers-Aris CA. Determination of a maximum number of artificial inseminations by donor children per sperm donor. Fertil Steril 1995;63:419–421
2. Curie-Cohen M. The frequency of consanguineous matings due to multiple use of donors in artificial insemination. Am J Hum Genet 1980;32:589–600
3. American College of Obstetricians and Gynecologists. Genetic screening for hemoglobinopathies. ACOG Committee Opinion 168. Washington, DC: ACOG, 1996

Bibliography

American College of Obstetricians and Gynecologists. Fragile X syndrome. ACOG Committee Opinion 161. Washington, DC: ACOG, 1995

American College of Obstetricians and Gynecologists. Hemoglobinopathies in pregnancy. ACOG Technical Bulletin 220. Washington, DC: ACOG, 1996

American College of Obstetricians and Gynecologists. Screening for Tay–Sachs disease. ACOG Committee Opinion 162. Washington, DC: ACOG, 1995

ASRM guidelines for gamete donation: 1993. Fertil Steril 1993;59(2 suppl 1):1S–9S

Barrat CL, Matson DL, Holt W. British Andrology Society guidelines for the screening of semen donors for donor insemination. Hum Reprod 1993;8:1521–1523

Curie-Cohen M, Luttrell L, Shapiro S. Current practice of artificial insemination by donor in the United States. N Engl J Med 1979;300:585–590

Findlay I, Cuckle H, Lilford RJ, Rutherford AJ, Quirke P, Lui S. Screening sperm donors for cystic fibrosis. BMJ 1995; 310:1533

Fraser FC, Forse RA. On genetic screening of donors for artificial insemination. Am J Med Genet 1981;10:399–405

Greiss MA, Terry P, Urbaniak SJ. Artificial insemination in RhD negative women. Hum Reprod 1995;10:2176

Jalbert P, Leonard C, Selva J, David G. Genetic aspects of artificial insemination with donor semen: the French CECOS Federation Guidelines. Am J Med Genet 1989;33:369–375

Modell B. Ethical aspects of genetic screening. Ann Med 1992;24:549–555

Pierce J, Reitemeier PJ, Jameton A, Maclin VM, DeJonge CJ. Should gamete donation between family members be restricted? The case of a 16-year-old donor. Hum Reprod 1995; 10:1330–1337

Smith PE. Selection against genetic defects in semen donors. Clin Genet 1984;26:87–108

Van Steirteghem AC, Pados G, Devroey P, Bonduelle M, Van Assche E, Liebaers I. Oocyte donation for genetic indications. Reprod Fertil Dev 1992;4:681–688

Wood EC. Oocyte donation—recent trends and concerns. Med J Aust 1994;160:282–284

ACOG Committee Opinion

Committee on Genetics

Number 230, January 2000

Maternal Phenylketonuria

Phenylketonuria (PKU) is an autosomal recessive disorder of phenylalanine metabolism that, if untreated, can cause severe mental retardation. Phenylketonuria is caused by a deficiency of the enzyme phenylalanine hydroxylase. Children of women with PKU will carry at least one abnormal gene, which is inherited from their homozygous affected mother. Even though the fetus is unlikely to be affected, approximately 1 in 120 children will inherit an abnormal phenylalanine hydroxylase gene from both parents and also have PKU. The remainder of children are carriers and should receive genetic counseling in the future. Phenylalanine crosses the placenta by an active transport process that results in a fetal-to-maternal plasma phenylalanine ratio of 1.5. This results in higher levels of phenylalanine in fetal blood than would be expected based on maternal blood levels.

Routine screening for PKU in newborns and early dietary therapy with a phenylalanine-restricted diet have markedly reduced mental retardation in affected individuals. As a result of these advances in the detection and treatment of PKU, there are large numbers of young adults with PKU who received early dietary treatment for this disorder and have IQs in the normal or near-normal range. The failure of young women with PKU to adhere to dietary restrictions has led to a new public health challenge. The heterozygous fetus is metabolically normal. However, these metabolically normal fetuses of women with PKU who are on an unrestricted diet may develop microcephaly, low birth weight, heart defects, and mental retardation due to maternal hyperphenylalaninemia. Children of women with PKU on unrestricted diets are at a 92% risk for mental retardation, a 73% risk for microcephaly, and a 12% risk for congenital heart defects (1).

In the United States, approximately 3,000 women of reproductive age are affected with PKU. Evidence indicates that women with PKU will benefit from remaining on a phenylalanine-free diet throughout their lives. Many of these women are not currently on phenylalanine-restricted diets, which require the consumption of phenylalanine-free products and supplements that many women find unpalatable. Unless these women are identified and placed on an appropriate diet before and during pregnancy, they are at risk for having children affected with PKU. It has been suggested that dietary control should be implemented at least 3 months prior to conception to help prevent fetal structural defects, including cardiac defects (2). If phenylalanine levels are normalized by 8 weeks of gestation, there is evidence to suggest a reduction in intrauterine growth restriction (3).

ISSN 1074-861X

The American College of Obstetricians and Gynecologists
409 12th Street, SW
PO Box 96920
Washington, DC 20090-6920

Conclusions and Recommendations

1. All women with PKU should be strongly encouraged to receive family planning and preconceptional counseling.
2. Women with PKU should begin dietary phenylalanine restriction prior to conception (4).
3. Ideally, pregnant women with PKU should be managed in consultation with practitioners from experienced PKU centers.

References

1. Lenke RR, Levy HL. Maternal phenylketonuria and hyperphenylalaninemia. An international survey of the outcome of untreated and treated pregnancies. N Engl J Med 1980; 303:1202–1208
2. Waisbren SE, Hamilton BD, St. James PJ, Shiloh S, Levy HL. Psychosocial factors in maternal phenylketonuria: women's adherence to medical recommendations. Am J Public Health 1995;85:1636–1641
3. Koch R, Friedman E, Azen C, Hanley W, Levy H, Matalon R, et al. The international collaborative study of maternal phenylketonuria status report 1998. MRDD Res Rev 1999;5:117–121
4. Levy HL, Waisbren SE, Lobbregt D, Allred E, Schuler A, Trefz FK, et al. Maternal mild hyperphenylalaninaemia: an international survey of offspring outcome. Lancet 1994; 344:1589–1594

Bibliography

Koch R, Levy HL, Matalon R, Rouse B, Haney WB, Trefz F, et al. The international collaborative study of maternal phenylketonuria: status report 1994. Acta Paediatr Suppl 1994;407: 111–119

Levy HL, Waisbren SE. Effects of untreated maternal phenylketonuria and hyperphenylalaninemia on the fetus. N Engl J Med 1983;309:1269–1274

Lipson A, Beuhler B, Bartley J, Walsh D, Yu J, O'Halloran M, et al. Maternal hyperphenylalaninemia fetal effects. J Pediatr 1984;104:216–220

Luke B, Keith LG. The challenge of maternal phenylketonuria screening and treatment. J Reprod Med 1990;35:667–673

MacCready RA. Admissions of phenylketonuric patients to residential institutions before and after screening programs of the newborn infant. J Pediatr 1974;85:383–385

Platt LD, Koch R, Azen C, Hanley WB, Levy HL, Matalon R, et al. Maternal phenylketonuria collaborative study, obstetric aspects and outcome: the first 6 years. Am J Obstet Gynecol 1992;166:1150–1162

ACOG

Committee on
Obstetric Practice

Committee
on Genetics

Committee Opinion

Number 183, April 1997

Routine Storage of Umbilical Cord Blood for Potential Future Transplantation

Reconstitution of the bone marrow can be a life-saving procedure in the treatment of hematologic disease (eg, Fanconi anemia) or advanced malignancy. The necessary hematopoietic stem and progenitor cells are usually obtained from allogeneic or autologous bone marrow. If autologous marrow is not an option, then a human leukocyte antigen (HLA)-identical sibling is the donor most likely to result in successful engraftment and minimization of the risk of graft-versus-host (GVH) disease. Most people do not have an HLA-identical sibling available, and they must look outside of their families. There is a national registry of potential bone marrow donors, but finding an identical match and convincing that individual to undergo the unpleasant donation procedure is not always easy. Many individuals who could potentially benefit from transplantation die while awaiting donors.

A recently recognized potential source for hematopoietic stem and progenitor cells is human fetal cord blood. Early results from more than 200 transplants of human cord stem cells, primarily to treat childhood malignancies, seem very encouraging for several reasons. There appears to be a relatively high success rate for the procedure even in the face of HLA mismatches at one or more loci. There also appears to be a somewhat lower risk for GVH disease than that which is true for traditional bone marrow transplantation. These encouraging preliminary reports have generated considerable enthusiasm because the 4 million births per year in the United States would appear to provide a large reservoir of genetically diverse, potentially transplantable specimens. Large volumes of cord blood are now being "wasted" as "discarded human material" that could theoretically be easily collected, typed, screened for infections, and banked cryogenically for transplantation.

The use of this technology raises a number of scientific, legal, and ethical issues that need to be addressed:

- Should cord blood specimens be collected and banked centrally for allogeneic transplantation in a system analogous to the way that we now handle blood, or would parents be well-advised to bank their own child's cord blood at birth for potential future autologous use should it ever be necessary?

ISSN 1074-861X

The American College of Obstetricians and Gynecologists
409 12th Street, SW
PO Box 96920
Washington, DC 20090-6920

- What is the probability that any individual will ever need his or her own cord blood for transplantation? If that need does arise 18 years later, what is the probability that a specimen stored for 18 years will still be viable?
- Most transplants to date have been done in babies and young children. More cells are needed to reconstitute the bone marrow of persons of larger size. What percentage of cord blood specimens will have adequate numbers of cells to reconstitute the bone marrow of adults?
- Are cord blood stem and progenitor cells more efficient at reconstituting marrow than are cells obtained from adult marrow? Would fewer cells on a per-kilogram body weight basis be as effective?
- Could the number of stem and progenitor cells in a specimen of cord blood be expanded in vitro to provide enough cells for a reliable reconstitution of the bone marrow of persons of adult size?
- If the apparently lower incidence of GVH disease compared with adult marrow sources is real, it may represent reduced immunocompetence of cord stem and progenitor cells. This may be disadvantageous in treating patients with cancer. It may also permit a higher incidence of second primary cancers in transplant survivors.
- As many as 38% of cord blood specimens may be contaminated with maternal cells. What effect will this contamination with adult cells that are (presumably) immunocompetent have upon graft success rate?
- In the future, there may be other medical approaches to manage these diseases.
- Should this technology continue to show promise, and the decision is made to establish cord blood banks, should cord blood continue to be regarded as "discarded human material?"
- Could cord blood be collected routinely at deliveries without consent?
- All specimens would need to be tested for infectious and selected genetic diseases before use. Should parents be informed if their child's specimen tests positive for an infection (eg, human immunodeficiency virus) or genetic disease?
- If nonpaternity is discovered in the course of testing, should that be disclosed to the mother, father, or child?
- Physicians should resist the pressures of marketing, and they should evaluate thoroughly the potential benefits and risks—emotional as well as physical—of all new medical interventions.

Privately owned for-profit companies have been established to bank cord blood samples for potential future use by those individuals or their family members. There is a significant cost associated with the initial specimen processing (approximately $1,500) and an annual storage fee (approximately $100). Given the low probability of needing a stem cell transplant (which has been estimated at between 1 in 1,000 and 1 in 200,000 by age 18) and the other uncertainties regarding success rates with increasing body mass and time in storage, is this a "good" investment? In view of the apparent success rate, despite HLA mismatch, will there be an advantage to receiving one's own banked cells, or could one do just as well with someone else's cord blood? Once banked, to whom do the cells there belong? Do they belong to the parents who paid the fees or the child from whom they came? Do the parents have the right to give them away or sell them, or should they be held for the person from whom they came until he or she reaches the age of majority? If the cells are to be used for someone other than the person from whom they came, must both parents agree or is consent from one adequate? What happens if the parents disagree?

There are clearly many questions about this technology that remain to be answered. Some are relatively simple, such as the success rate of the procedure for various diseases and at various body weights. These simply await a larger number of cases. Some will be more difficult, such as the viability of cells in long-term storage; these questions will take time to answer. The most difficult will be the moral, ethical, and social questions, which need extensive public discussion and may never all be resolved to everyone's satisfaction. Until there is a fuller understanding of all of these issues, we must proceed with considerable circumspection. Parents should not be sold this service without a realistic assessment of their likely return on their investment. Commercial cord blood banks should not represent the service they sell as "doing everything possible" to ensure the health of children. Parents and grandparents should not be made to feel guilty if they are not eager or able to invest these considerable sums in such a highly speculative venture.

Bibliography

Broxmeyer HE. Questions to be answered regarding umbilical cord blood hematopoietic stem and progenitor cells and their use in transplantation. Transfusion 1995;35:694-702

Kurtzberg J, Laughlin M, Graham ML, Smith C, Olson JF, Halperin EC, et al. Placental blood as a source of hematopoietic stem cells for transplantation into unrelated recipients. N Engl J Med 1996;335:157-166

Laporte JP, Gorin NC, Rubinstein P, Lesage S, Portnoi MF, Barbu V, et al. Cord-blood transplantation from an unrelated donor in an adult with chronic myelogenous leukemia. N Engl J Med 1996;335:167-170

Marshall E. Clinical promise, ethical quandary. Science 1996;271:586-588

Rubinstein P, Rosenfield RE, Adamson JW, Stevens CE. Stored placental blood for unrelated bone marrow reconstitution. Blood 1993;81:1679-1690

Scaradavou A, Carrier C, Mollen N, Stevens C, Rubenstein P. Detection of maternal DNA in placental/umbilical cord blood by locus-specific amplification of the noninherited maternal HLA gene. Blood 1996;88:1494-1500

Silberstein LE, Jefferies LC. Placental-blood banking—a new frontier in transfusion medicine. N Engl J Med 1996;335:199-201

Wagner JE, Rosenthal J, Sweetman R, Shu XO, Davies SM, Ramsay NK, et al. Successful transplantation of HLA-matched and HLA-mismatched umbilical cord blood from unrelated donors: analysis of engraftment and acute graft-versus-host disease. Blood 1996:88:795-802

ACOG

Committee on Genetics

Committee Opinion

Number 212, November 1998

Screening for Canavan Disease

Canavan disease is a severe progressive genetic disorder of the central nervous system. The clinical features of Canavan disease usually appear after the first few months of life and include developmental delay, macrocephaly, hypotonia, and poor head control. As the disease progresses, seizures, optic atrophy, gastrointestinal reflux, and deterioration of swallowing develop. Most children with Canavan disease die in the first decade of life. Presently, there is no cure or effective therapy for Canavan disease.

Canavan disease is caused by a deficiency of the enzyme aspartoacylase, which leads to increased excretion of its substrate, *N*-acetylaspartic acid (NAA). A diagnosis of Canavan disease is established by determining an increased level of urinary NAA by organic acid analysis. These abnormally high levels of NAA lead to demyelination and spongy degeneration of the brain, which cause the neurologic features of Canavan disease.

As in Tay–Sachs disease, Canavan disease is inherited as an autosomal recessive condition and is more prevalent among individuals of Eastern European Jewish (Ashkenazi) background. It is estimated that the carrier frequency in the Ashkenazi Jewish population is approximately 1 per 40. Thus, the risk for an affected offspring in this population approximates 1 in 6,400 births. Unlike Tay–Sachs disease, however, there do not appear to be other high-risk ethnic populations, although Canavan disease has been reported in individuals of non-Ashkenazi Jewish background.

Molecular studies have revealed two specific mutations in the aspartoacylase gene on chromosome 17. These account for approximately 97% of the mutations causing Canavan disease in the Ashkenazi Jewish population. One is a mutation in codon 285 of the aspartoacylase gene, and the other is a mutation in codon 231. Screening of Ashkenazi Jewish individuals can be performed by analyzing for these two mutations. In non-Jewish persons, the mutations may be different and more diverse. The most common mutation is in codon 305, which has been noted in approximately 36% of the 70 identified alleles from unrelated non-Jewish individuals.

Carrier screening for Canavan disease requires molecular diagnostic methods. Simple enzymatic assays, as commonly used in Tay–Sachs screening, cannot be used for Canavan disease because the activity of the deficient enzyme, aspartoacylase, is not detectable in blood. Testing for the three most common Canavan disease mutations will identify about 97% of Ashkenazi Jewish carriers and 40–50% of non-Jewish carriers.

ISSN 1074-861X

The American College of Obstetricians and Gynecologists
409 12th Street, SW
PO Box 96920
Washington, DC 20090-6920

When both parents are carriers of identifiable Canavan disease mutations, prenatal diagnosis by chorionic villus sampling (CVS) or amniocentesis can be accomplished using DNA analysis. In couples where one or both members have unknown mutations, biochemical analysis of NAA levels in the amniotic fluid can be used reliably. Elevated NAA levels can be used to detect an affected fetus. The analysis should be done in a laboratory that has personnel who have expertise in performing this test. Enzyme analysis of aspartoacylase in cultured fetal cells from CVS or amniocentesis is not reliable.

Based on the preceding information, the Committee on Genetics makes the following recommendations:

1. Ideally, molecular carrier screening for Canavan disease should be offered preconceptionally if both members of the couple are of Ashkenazi Jewish genetic background. This screening could be combined with screening for Tay–Sachs disease because both disorders are more common in this group. Many specialized laboratories already offer screening for both diseases. Those with a family history consistent with Canavan disease also should be offered screening, which should be voluntary; informed consent and assurance of confidentiality are required. If potential carriers have not been screened preconceptionally, screening may be offered during early pregnancy.
2. If only one partner is of high risk (of Ashkenazi Jewish descent or with a family history consistent with Canavan disease), this partner should be screened first. Ideally, this should be performed preconceptionally. If it is determined that the high-risk partner is a carrier, the other partner should be offered screening. The couple, however, must be informed of the limitations of testing. If the woman is already pregnant, it may be necessary to screen both partners simultaneously so that results are obtained in a timely fashion and to ensure that all options are available for the couple.
3. If it is determined by DNA-based analysis that both partners are carriers of Canavan disease, prenatal diagnosis should be offered either by CVS or amniocentesis, using DNA-based testing of the fetal cells.

Bibliography

American College of Medical Genetics Board of Directors. Position statement on carrier testing for Canavan disease. Bethesda, Maryland: January 10, 1998

American College of Obstetricians and Gynecologists. Screening for Tay–Sachs disease. ACOG Committee Opinion 162. Washington, DC: ACOG, 1995

Bennett MJ, Gibson KM, Sherwood WG, Divry P, Rolland MO, Elpeleg ON, et al. Reliable prenatal diagnosis of Canavan disease (aspartoacylase deficiency): comparison of enzymatic and metabolite analysis. J Inherit Metab Dis 1993;16:831–836

Kaul R, Gao GP, Matalon M, Aloya M, Su Q, Jin M, et al. Identification and expression of eight novel mutations among non-Jewish patients with Canavan disease. Am J Hum Genet 1996;59:95–102

Kronn D, Oddoux C, Philips J, Ostrer H. Prevalence of Canavan disease heterozygotes in the New York metropolitan Ashkenazi Jewish population. Am J Hum Genet 1995;57:1250–1252

Matalon R. Canavan disease: diagnosis and molecular analysis. Genetic Testing 1997;1:21–25

Matalon R, Michals K, Kaul R. Canavan disease: from spongy degeneration to molecular analysis. J Pediatr 1995;127:511–517

ACOG

Committee on Genetics

Committee Opinion

Number 162, November 1995 *(Replaces #93, March 1991)*

Screening for Tay–Sachs Disease

Tay–Sachs Disease (TSD) is a lysosomal storage disease in which GM_2 gangliosides accumulate throughout the body. The accumulation of these gangliosides in the central nervous system results in a severe progressive neurologic disease with death in early childhood.

The enzyme hexosaminidase occurs in two principal forms, Hex-A and Hex-B. Hex-A is composed of one α- and one β-subunit, whereas Hex-B is composed of two β-subunits. Tay–Sachs disease is caused by a deficiency of Hex-A, whereas Sandhoff disease is caused by a deficiency of both Hex-A and Hex-B. Both of these diseases are transmitted in an autosomal recessive fashion. Laboratories report Hex-A levels as a percentage of total hexosaminidase activity. Hex-A is almost completely absent in patients with classical TSD. Hex-A comprises 0.5% of total hexosaminidase activity in the late infantile type and 2–4% in the adult form activity. The percentage of Hex-A activity in carriers is usually less than 55% of total activity, whereas Hex-A activity in non-carriers is generally more than 60% of total activity. Tay–Sachs disease can be diagnosed prenatally by measuring hexosaminidase activity in samples obtained by amniocentesis or by chorionic villus sampling.

The frequency of TSD carriers in Jews of Eastern European descent (Ashkenazi) is about 1 in 30; the carrier rate for non-Jewish groups is estimated at 1 in 300. It has been determined that people of French–Canadian and Cajun descent also have a greater carrier frequency than the general population.

Carrier screening using serum is inaccurate when performed in women who are pregnant or taking oral contraceptives. If the serum test is used, many pregnant women will be misclassified as carriers. If testing is to be done in women who are pregnant or taking oral contraceptives, leukocyte testing must be used.

Molecular analyses of the α-subunit gene for TSD have been reported in both Jewish and non-Jewish populations. Three mutations comprise more than 90% of mutant genes in Ashkenazi Jewish persons. Other less common mutations are often seen in non-Jewish carriers. Molecular analysis may be required in some of these patients.

When the serum test is inconclusive, biochemical analysis should be performed on leukocytes from peripheral blood. DNA analysis is reserved for those couples who consistently have ambiguous enzymatic tests in both

ISSN 1074-861X

The American College of Obstetricians and Gynecologists
409 12th Street, SW
Washington, DC 20024-2188

serum and leukocytes and for individuals who are suspected to have a rare pseudodeficiency condition.

Pseudodeficiency refers to a state in which asymptomatic individuals have a low amount of Hex-A activity when tested with conventional artificial substrate. However, these normal but Hex-A–minus individuals are able to catalyze the breakdown of natural substrate GM_2 ganglioside. Pseudodeficiency mutations comprise about one third of the mutations identified in non-Jewish individuals. Because some of these individuals are compound heterozygotes for a Tay–Sachs mutation and a pseudodeficiency allele, the delineation of their precise genotype for reproductive purposes usually requires further biochemical assessment complemented with DNA analysis.

Based on the preceding information, the Committee on Genetics makes the following recommendations:

1. Ideally, serum screening for TSD should be offered before pregnancy if both members of a couple are Ashkenazi Jews or of French–Canadian or Cajun descent. Those with a family history consistent with TSD should also be screened.
2. When one member of a couple is at high risk (ie, Ashkenazi Jew, of French–Canadian or Cajun descent, or has a family history consistent with TSD) but the other partner is not, the high-risk partner should be screened. This is particularly important if there is uncertainty about ancestry or if there is a family history consistent with TSD. If the high-risk partner is determined to be a carrier, the other partner should also be screened. If the woman is already pregnant, it may be necessary to screen both partners simultaneously so that results are obtained in a timely fashion and to ensure that all options are available to the couple.
3. Ambiguous screening tests or positive screening tests in individuals not at high risk should be confirmed by molecular analysis for the most common mutations. This will detect patients who carry genes associated with mild disease or pseudodeficiency states.
4. If TSD screening is performed in women who are pregnant or on oral contraceptives, leukocyte testing must be used.
5. If both partners are determined to be carriers of TSD, genetic counseling and prenatal diagnosis should be offered (1).

Reference

1. American College of Obstetricians and Gynecologists. Antenatal diagnosis of genetic disorders. ACOG Technical Bulletin 108. Washington, DC: ACOG, 1987

Bibliography

Kaback M, Lim-Steele J, Dabholkar D, Brown D, Levy N, Zeiger K. Tay-Sachs disease—carrier screening, prenatal diagnosis, and the molecular era. An international perspective, 1970 to 1993. The International TSD Data Collection Network. JAMA 1993;270:2307–2315

Prence EM, Natowicz MR, Zalewski I. Unusual thermolability properties of leukocyte beta-hexosaminidase: implications in screening for carriers of Tay-Sachs disease. Clin Chem 1993; 39:1811–1814

Triggs-Raine BL, Feigenbaum AS, Natowicz M, Skomorowski MA, Schuster SM, Clarke JT, et al. Screening for carriers of Tay-Sachs disease among Ashkenazi Jews. A comparison of DNA-based and enzyme-based tests. N Engl J Med 1990; 32:6–12

Index

Note: Page numbers followed by italicized letters *f* and *t* indicate figures and tables, respectively.